Essays in Medical Biography

Essays in Medical Biography

J. T. Hughes

Rimes House
Oxford
2008

British Library Cataloguing in Publication Data
A catalogue record for this book is available from the British Library.

     Essays in Medical Biography
     Hughes, J.T. 1928-

1. Biography. 2. Medical History. 3. 17th Century Science.

ISBN 978-1-874317-01-2

Typeset in Sabon and printed by
The Holywell Press Ltd.
15-17 Kings Meadow
Ferry Hinksey Road
Oxford OX2 0DP

ACKNOWLEDGEMENTS

SIXTEEN OF THESE essays have appeared in medical and historical journals and, for their reproduction, I am grateful to the editors and publishers of the following: *Scottish Medical Journal, Cheshire History, The London Journal, Yorkshire History Quarterly, Norfolk Archaeology, Transactions of the Halifax Antiquarian Society, Journal of Neurology*, and the *Journal of Medical Biography*. I am especially indebted to Dr Christopher Gardner-Thorpe, editor of the *Journal of Medical Biography*, where seven of these essays appeared and to Dr John A Hargreaves who published the three articles in the *Transactions of the Halifax Antiquary Society*, and has given permission on behalf of the Society. Articles eleven and twelve appeared as chapters of books, to whose editors and publishers I record my thanks. Each individual reference appears after the title in the list of contents. For illustrations, I am grateful to libraries, record offices, and individuals. My especial thanks are to the Bodleian Library and the British Library for the assistance of their staff over many years. The National Portrait Gallery have provided portraits of Sir William Petty and Laurence Sterne.

I am indebted to many other libraries and record depositories and would mention those of London (the Library of the Royal College of Physicians, the Library of the Royal Society, the Guildhall Library, and the Wellcome Library), Chester (the Chester City Record Office and the Cheshire Record Office), Halifax (The Halifax Central Library), Norwich (The Norfolk Record Office), Swindon (The National Monuments Record) and York (The Borthwick Institute of Historical Research). The staff of the Library of the Faculty of Medicine of Montpellier facilitated the research described in chapters 1 and 4.

The expert work of Ben Burrows, Trevor Pratt, and Rachel James of the Holywell Press has created this book from a miscellany of printed scripts and assorted memory discs.

Throughout my 50 years in Oxford, my career in medical research has been accompanied by an interest in history fostered by contact with the historians of Oxford. Some have been personal friends and have encouraged the writing of these essays. Hugh Trevor Roper, Robert Blake and Jennifer Loach are now only in memory, but Barbara Harvey, Keith Thomas, Peter Mathias, and Charles Webster are still active. All these historians have seen one or more of these essays, which however fall far short of their products. My final thanks are to my wife, Catherine, who has cast a historian's eye over all these essays and encouraged their publication.

Green College
University of Oxford, Woodstock Road
Oxford OX2 6HG

CONTENTS

LIST OF ILLUSTRATIONS

George Scharpe, c.1581-1637
A Scots Doctor at Montpellier

Abstract: Before the eighteenth century many Scots studied medicine at the medical schools of Europe, of which Montpellier was frequently the choice. George Scharpe, an early student of the University of Edinburgh, graduated in medicine at Montpellier and joined the medical faculty, where his long career can be traced from contemporary records. The practice of Scots studying abroad is described, as is Languedoc in the early seventeenth century – a region and period devastated by the religious wars of France.

Key words: George Scharpe, Scots physicians abroad, University of Montpellier, Languedoc, French religious wars

In the fifteenth century, three universities were founded in Scotland: St Andrew's (1413), Glasgow (1451), and Aberdeen (1494).[1] All were church foundations initiated by scholars and senior clerics of these towns, and authorised by the Pope. One or more Papal Bulls directed the King of Scotland to pass the required statutes. Enterprising Scots students still sought tuition in the universities of France, Italy[2], Germany and sometimes further afield, but gradually higher education was established locally.[3]

Then came the reformation in Scotland. In 1559-1560, the Scots Parliament abolished Papal authority and adopted the Protestant 'Confession of Faith'. The three universities were forced to comply, Aberdeen with reluctance, St. Andrew's and Glasgow with more enthusiasm.[4] The reformation saved the older universities, which were failing mainly from confining their teaching to theology. There were few pupils: the English Ambassador in Scotland, writing in 1562, described only 'fifteen or sixteen scollers' at Aberdeen.[5] Thus came the foundation of a protestant university in the capital, encouraged, amongst others by James Lawson, a local minister, who, in 1578, presented a petition to James VI. A charter to found the University was granted in 1580.[6] Though only fourteen years of age, the King, well taught in Latin and Greek, and versed in Calvinist theology, welcomed the University in the words 'I will be godfather to the College of Edinburgh and will have it called the College of King James'.[7] The official title was *Academi Jacobi Sexti*. There was a link between the King and Languedoc, of which Montpellier was the famous seat of learning. James eventually married Anne of Denmark, but there had been an alternate bride in Catherine de Bourbon, sister of Henry of Navarre, of whom we shall hear later. Catherine – a French princess – had the distinction of being Huguenot and Calvinist.

1

Whilst students could now study in Scotland, many subsequently visited the continent, where they were welcome, and some remained to teach. Of Bordeaux University, Vinetus wrote 'This school is rarely without a Scotsman; it has two at present – one of whom is a professor of philosophy, the other of the Greek language and mathematics...'.[8] These two professors were William Hegate and Robert Balfour. John Cameron, 1580-1625, was described as a 'vagrant Scottish scholar, filling successively a chair in half the universities of western Europe'.[9] In medicine, although Paris attracted pupils, the Universities of Montpellier, Padua, and Leiden were successively famous. Montpellier, the oldest surviving medical school in Europe, attracted scholars in the sixteenth century and earlier; by 1600 Padua was more favoured; and by the end of the seventeenth century, tuition at Leiden was the most coveted.[10] A notable example of a Scots doctor abroad was George Scharpe (Figure 1.1), who, coming to Montpellier for his medical studies, remained there for almost the whole of his career.[11]

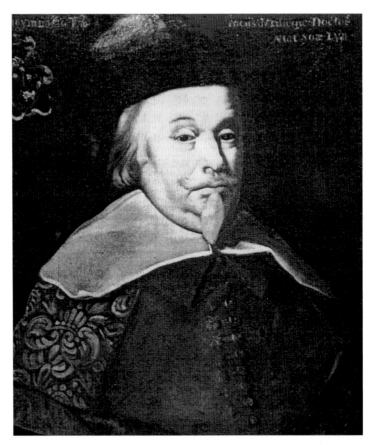

Figure 1.1 George Scharpe. Reproduced,with permission, from Dulieu L. *La Médicine á Montpellier, Avingnon, Les Presses Universelles*, 1975–1990, 3, (2), 642. The original is an oil painting in the Faculty of Medicine of Montpellier.

Scharpe at Edinburgh

Scharpe was a product of the University of Edinburgh where he began his studies
in the autumn of 1596. He graduated among 32 in the 13th class on 29 July, 1600,
under John Adamson, Regent.[12] Mr Robert Rollack, a Minister in the City, had
been Principal of the new College for 15 years – almost from its foundation – but
died in February 1599, to be succeeded the following year by Mr Henry Charteris.
Other teachers in Scharpe's time included Charles Ferme (to 1598), George
Robertson (to 1598), William Crage, John Roy, and Robert Scot.[13]

The curriculum for attaining the Master of Arts degree had been designed in
1583.[14] There were four years or classes, the first being the 'Bajan' class[15] in which
Latin and Greek predominated, texts being Cicero, Clenardus (a Greek grammar),
the New Testament, and Homer *etc*. The second, or Semi-Bajan year, studied
further classics, particularly Aristotle, but were also instructed in Rhetoric and
Arithmetic. Disputation now formed a common mode of instruction. In the third
or Bachelor year, Hebrew, Dialectics, and Human Anatomy were added. The final,
or Magistrand year, repeated previous work but added Practical Astronomy,
Meteorology, and Cosmography (geography).

Edinburgh was experiencing changes during this period.[16] The King came to
reside in the City, and there was interest in his marriage to Anne of Denmark. Anne
was stormbound in Oslo, whither James sailed in November 1589, to marry his
Queen, and bring her to Edinburgh in May 1590.

Medical tuition at Montpellier

Edinburgh University was not to develop a medical school untill the last quarter of
the seventeenth century. To pursue his medical studies, Scharpe proceeded to the
University of Montpellier, the oldest medical school in Europe, and whose history
has been much researched.[17] [18] [19] [20]

An early narrative is that of Jean Astruc. We are indebted to Louis Dulieu for a
comprehensive modern account, which gathers many contemporary records. The
medical archives, together with a collection of works on the history of the medical
school, are in the Faculty of Medicine Library. I am grateful to the Faculty of
Medicine for permission to peruse these archives and publications.

Scharpe's choice of medical school was probably determined by religion:
Edinburgh was Calvinist, as was Montpellier. At this time, whilst the main part of
France was Catholic, some of the towns in the south were protestant, of which
Montpellier was one. The majority of the population were protestants who
dominated civic affairs and filled the chairs of the University. Montpellier was
favoured by the friendship of the king, Henry IV, whose early life was spent in this
area. Henry (of Navarre) was brought up by his mother as a Calvinist, and was the
leader in the third Huguenot war, in which, however, he lost the battle of Jarnac
in 1569. The murder of Henry, Duke of Guise, by Henry III, who himself was

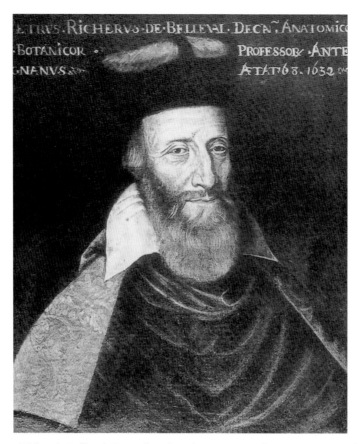

Figure 1.2 Pierre Richer de Bellaval. Reproduced, with permission, from *Rioux J-A. ed. Le Jardin des Plantes de Montpellier, Graulhet Cedex, Editions Odyssée*, 1994, 25. The original is an oil painting in the Faculty of Medicine of Montpellier.

murdered, brought the crown to Henry of Navarre, now Henry IV. Evidence of the King's interest in the university and in the medical school was his founding, in 1593, of the Jardin des Plantes, the first academic botanical garden in France, with two supportive chairs of anatomy and botany.[21]

Scharpe[22] arrived in Montpellier in 1601 to study 'belles-lettres' in the faculty of arts under the Protestant Chair of Philosophy.[23] His medical studies began with his matriculation on October 30th 1603.[24] Pierre Richer de Bellaval[25] (Figure 1.2), 1564-1632, was the senior physician, first Director of the Botanic Garden, and Professor of Anatomy and of Botany, a frequent combination.[26] Pierre's colleagues in teaching Scharpe were Jean Varanda, Professor of Medicine[27] and Pierre Dortoman, Professor of Surgery and Pharmacy.[28] After 1605, Surgery and Pharmacy were separated: Francois Ranchin became professor of surgery[29], whilst Dortoman remained Professor of Pharmacy. Another important position, occupied by Jacques d'Estienne de Pradilles[30], was that of physician to the poor hospital, L'Hotel- Dieu Saint-Eloi. Jacques was succeeded in 1604 by Pierre Dortoman, who in 1606 was replaced by Jacques de L'Hostallier.[31] All these academics were practising physicians and formed a strong academic team. The buildings in which they taught in the seventeenth century (Figure 1.3) were researched by Bonnet.[32]

Scharpe joins the Faculty

Scharpe graduated bachelor of medicine on January 13th, 1606, and on April 8th was licensed in medicine.[33] During 1607, 1608, and 1609, he was the physician in charge of the poor at *l'Hotel-Dieu Saint-Eloi*, displacing de L'Hostallier. On February 8th 1607, Scharpe obtained his doctorate in medicine, examined by Pierre Dortoman.[34] He presented a thesis entitled '*Questiones Medicae*'.[35] This was one of eight medical theses published in Montpellier in 1617; unfortunately no copy is known to have survived. [36] [37] Another, on carcinoma of the breast, was by a compatriot, Adam Abernethy.[38] In 1613, Scharpe taught in the botanic garden as a demonstrator of 'simples'.[39] By now his work was respected and, in 1619, he was made 'Regence IV'.[40] He was appointed in 1619 to the chair of

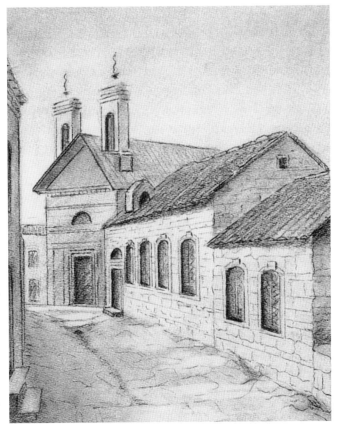

Figure 1.3 The Medical School in Montpellier in the 17th century. Drawing based on research by Hubert Bonnet. Reproduced, with permission from Bonnet H. *La Faculté de Medicine de Montpellier, Sauramps Medical*, 1992, 13.

medicine, made vacant by the death of Jean Varanda in 1617. There was strong competition, one unsuccessful applicant being Lazarre Rivière, later to prove an outstanding physician at Montpellier.[41]   In 1618 and 1619 Scharpe taught Pharmacy to apprentice apothecaries.[42]   He was now married to Francoise de la Combe, a Protestant lady of Montpellier and, of several children, the sons, Claude, Jacques, and Jules-Georges, were destined for medicine in Montpellier. Scharpe's seniority in the Faculty was now evident. He was made Proctor in 1631, and Vice-Chancellor in 1632, in the absence of Francois Ranchin. He seems to have been difficult with colleagues, and as Proctor was quarrelsome and arrogant at examinations, for which, in 1631, he was threatened with a fine and a 'deposition'. He transgressed further and in 1634, at a faculty meeting, he called Pompee Andre, demonstrator in botany, an ignoramus. He and Jacques Duranc, a friend who supported Scharpe in this defiance, were censured. But Scharpe was soon to leave Montpellier.

To Bologna

Scharpe's fame attracted the Italian medical schools – Venice and Bologna – who sought his services. Bologna, the oldest of the Italian schools and one of the richest, enticed him to a chair created for him in the 'Theory of Medicine'. Also relevant was the desperate state of Montpellier at this time: see below. Scharpe departed for Bologna in 1634.[43]   He left the Faculty in confusion, as he nominated Jacques Duranc as his successor. This irregular appointment appalled the seniors of the medical school, who wished to appoint a candidate of their own choice. It seemed their right, but Scharpe proved wily and obstinate, arguing that the King had appointed him in Montpellier, and, as his move to Bologna might be temporary, he could appoint Duranc as his locum tenens. This unlikely liberty provoked legal challenge. An influential friend – M. de Fenouillet, Eveque of Montpellier – supported Scharpe, affirming that he had gone to Bologna, *Animo Redeundi*, with the permission of the King. The case was sent to Toulouse for trial, which promised not only controversy but scandal: it was alleged that Duranc had paid Scharpe for his appointment.[44] The Parliament at Toulouse declared the chair vacant but the legal wrangle continued, only ending with the death of Scharpe (Figure 1.4) in Bologna in 1637, on 24 August, the anniversary of his birth.[45] It seems that he died having embraced the Catholic Church.

Scharpe's son, Claude returned to medical studies at Montpellier and in September, 1638 obtained his doctorate.[46]   In the same year he published the lecture notes of his father under the title '*Institutiones Medicae*'.[47]   The book is rare even in France – there is no copy in Montpellier –, but there are two copies in North America.[48]   These lectures are the main evidence of Scharpe's medical standing, which did not approach the fame of Ranchin[49] or Rivière in medicine or of Pierre Richer de Bellaval[50] in botany. But Guy Patin, 1601-1672, in Paris, never

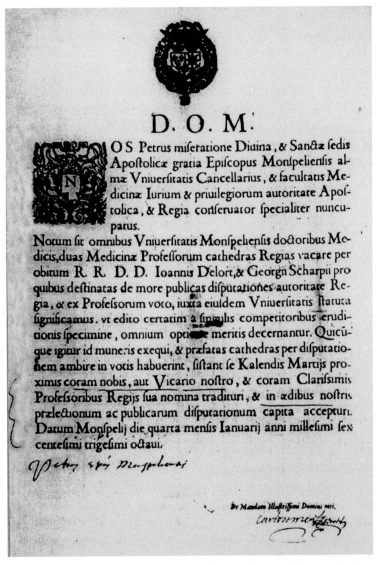

D. O. M.

OS Petrus miferatione Diuina, & Sanctæ fedis Apoftolicæ gratia Epifcopus Monfpelienfis almæ Vniuerfitatis Cancellarius, & facultatis Medicinæ Iurium & priuilegiorum autoritate Apoftolica, & Regia conferuator fpecialiter nuncupatus.

Notum fit omnibus Vniuerfitatis Monfpelienfis doctoribus Medicis, duas Medicinæ Profefforum cathedras Regias vacare per obitum R. R. D. D. Ioannis Delort, & Georgii Scharpii pro quibus deftinatas de more publicas difputationes autoritate Regia, & ex Profefforum voto, iuxta eiufdem Vniuerfitatis ftatuta fignificamus. vt edito certatim à fingulis competitoribus erudicionis fpecimine, omnium opti~ meritis decernantur. Quicúque igitur id muneris exequi, & præfatas cathedras per difputationem ambire in votis habuerint, fiftant fe Kalendis Martijs proximis coram nobis, aut Vicario noftro, & coram Clarifsimis Profefforibus Regijs fua nomina traditturi, & in ædibus noftris prælectionum ac publicarum difputationum capita accepturi. Datum Monfpelij die quarta menfis Ianuarij anni millefimi fex centefimi trigefimi octaui.

De Mandato Illuftiffimi Domini mei.

Figure 1.4 From the *Archives départmentales de l'Herault*: c.1324. Notice of the vacancy of two chairs arising from the deaths of Jean Derlot and George Scharpe. Reproduced, with permission from Dulieu, L. 3, (1), 46.

one to praise the physicians of Montpellier, considered Scharpe a very learned man and an able logician.[51]

The Religious Wars in France

During Scharpe's career in Montpellier – 1601 to 1634 –, much of the South of France was disturbed by a series of religious wars, the cause being the reformation as expressed by the Protestants or Hugenots.[52] The Hugenots were considered a threat to national unity. They formed only 5 to 6 per cent of the population of

France in the South but were numerous in some towns, notably, La Rochelle, but also Castres, Clairac, Millau, Montabaun, and Nerac which were wholly protestant. Henri IV had been a friend of the locality, and kindly disposed to Protestants, whose rights were recognised in 1598 by the Edict of Nantes, by which, in addition to religious freedom, Protestants had access to schools, universities, and hospitals. In Montpellier, they were in the majority, occupied most of the civic positions and the chairs in the University. Henry's assassination in 1610 ended this forbearance. There was an indecisive period when Marie de Medici, the mother of the child Louis XIII, was Regent, but when Louis assumed control in 1617, later aided, and almost supplanted by Cardinal Richelieu, war was declared on the Hugenots. As threatening as their religious incompabily, was their wealth and power in those towns they controlled. In 1628 La Rochelle surrendered after a prolonged siege, and the King and Cardinal turned further South, totally destroying many of the towns of Languedoc.[53] Louis laid siege to Montpellier in 1622[54], destroying most of the buildings of the town and devastating the celebrated *Jardin des Plantes*. The town surrendered on October 18th, 1622, in which year the 'Peace of Montpellier' was signed. Then followed a period of famine and epidemics. Significant is the prevalence of Morgellons, an illness now forgotten by the medical profession but associated with extreme poverty.[55] Plague came to Montpellier at the end of July, 1629, and, by November, 2000 inhabitants had died.[56] The epidemic abated in December and had ceased by February, 1630, by which time the towns of Pui, Carcassone, Montauban, and Toulouse were affected. The destruction of the city and the plague profoundly affected tuition in the medical school. The University Registers show the intake of medical students, usually over 30, reduced in 1629, when only 7 were matriculated. Numbers recovered the following year.

The physicians of the Montpellier medical school struggled through this disastrous period. First they were obliged to provide medical services to the protestant armies of Rohan.[57] Then, as best they could, they sheltered from the destruction of the town during the siege, and offered what medical assistance was possible. After the surrender, they began the reconstruction of the city and to cope with famine and sickness, notably the plague of 1629-1630. Prominent was Francois Ranchin, born and educated in Montpellier, Professor of Medicine since 1605, Chancellor in 1612, and author of many important texts.[58] Ranchin was active in the rebuilding of the city, including the hospitals, the medical school, and the anatomy theatre of Guillaume Rondelet.[59] Mayor of Montpellier during the plague of 1629-1630, Ranchin made great efforts to contain the epidemic and bring relief to the population. The other senior administrator, active in reconstuction, was his colleague, Pierre Richter de Belleval. Pierre had scarcely finished creating his beloved botanic garden when it was almost totally destroyed. In happier times, Henri IV had founded the garden. Now Pierre, without outside finance, set about its rebuilding and replanting, using his own fortune and that of his wife.[60] Untill he died in 1632, to be survived by his nephew, Martin Richer de Bellaval, all his resources were devoted to the garden and the building of a College of Botany.

In the records of the medical school there are references to Scharpe's services during these troubled years.[61] During the siege of 1622, he was directed to assist the soldiers of the Rohan, and later he visited those affected by the plague. But he did not see the full reconstruction of Montpellier and the recovery of the Medical School, as he left for Bologna in 1634.

ACKNOWLEDGEMENTS

I am grateful to the staffs of the Bodleian and British Libraries, the Library of the *Maison Francaise*, Oxford, and the Librarian and Archivist of the University of Montpellier. For the reproduction of figures, I thank the authors, publishers, and primary sources stated in the legends.

REFERENCES

1 Powicke, F.M. and Emden. A.B. Rashdall's Medieval Universities: *The Universities of Europe in the Middle Ages*. New edition in 3 volumes. Oxford, Clarendon Press, 1936, 2, 301-324.

2 Steuart, A.F. 'The Scottish 'Nation' at the University of Padua,' *Scottish History Revue*, 3. (1906); 53-62.

3 Dunlop, A.I. 'Scots Abroad in the Fifteenth Century,' *Historical Pamphlet No. 124*, London, Historical Association, P.S. King & Staples, 1942.

4 Grant, A. *The Story of the University of Edinburgh during its first Three Hundred Years*. In two vols. London, Longmans, Green & Co., 1884, 1, 50-53.

5 Grant, 1, 46.

6 Craufurd, T. *History of the University of Edinburgh from 1580 to 1646*, Edinburgh, A Neill & Co., 1808. Thomas Craufurd, Regent of Philosophy and Professor of Mathematics, died 1662, leaving the *ms.* which was published in 1808.

7 Grant, 1, 131.

8 Burton, J.H. *The Scot Abroad, Vols 1 & 2*, Edinburgh and London, W. Blackwood & Sons, 1864, 2, 103. *Vinetus* was Elie Vinet, 1509- 1587.

9 Irving, J. *The Book of Scotsmen*, Paisley, Alex Gardner, 1881, 57.

10 Hughes, J.T. 'The medical education of Sir Thomas Browne, a seventeenth-century student at Montpellier, Padua, and Leiden.' *Journal of Medical Biography*, 9 (2001), 70-76.

11 Short account, with errors, in : *Dictionary of National Biography*, Oxford, Oxford University Press, 1998, 17, 900-901.

12 *A Cataloque of the Graduates in the Faculty of Arts, Divinty, and Law of the University of Edinburgh since its foundation*, Edinburgh, Neill & Co, 1858, 17.

13 Craufurd, 38-53.

[14] Grant, 1, 144-150.

[15] The word 'Bajan' for a first year student comes from the University of Paris, Grant, 1, 145.

[16] Wilson, D. *Memorials of Edinburgh in the Olden Time*, Edinburgh: Adam & Charles Black, 1890-1891, 106-117.

[17] Astruc MJ. *Memoires pour servir à l'Histoire de La Faculte de médecine de Montpellier*, Paris: P.G. Cavelier, 1767.

[18] Germain, A.C. *L'Ecole de Médecine de Montpellier: Ses origenes, Sa Constitution, Son Enseignement*, Montpellier, J. Martel aine, 1880.

[19] Dulieu, L. *La Médecine à Montpellier*, vols. 1-4, Avignon: Les Presses Universelles, 1975-1990, the relevant volume, in two parts, being Tome 3, L'Epoque Classique (henceforth Dulieu).

[20] Bonnet, H. *La Faculte de Médecine de Montpellier*, Montpellier: Sauramps Medical, 1992.

[21] Rioux J-A. Ed. *Le Jardin des Plantes de Montpellier*, Graulhet Cedex: Editions Odyssee, 1994.

[22] Astruc, 255-256.

[23] Dulieu, 3, (2), 799.

[24] University of Montpellier, *Registers* (henceforth *Registers*), S. 20, f. 122 v. Reproduced in Dulieu, 3,(2), 745-755.

[25] Astruc, 253-254.

[26] Dulieu, 3, (2), 789-790.

[27] Dulieu, 3, (1), 26, 130, 150, and 196.

[28] Dulieu, 3, (2), 758-759.

[29] Dulieu, 3, (2), 785-786.

[30] Dulieu, 3, (2), 784.

[31] Dulieu, 3, (1), 561.

[32] Bonnet, 131.

[33] *Registers*, S.7, f.20, r.; Dulieu, 3, (2), 798-799.

[34] *Registers*, S.7, f.28, r-v, Dulieu, 3, (2), 789-790.

[35] Eloy, N.F.J. *Dictionnaire Historique de la Médecine Ancienne et Moderne*, Mons, H. Hoyois, 1778, 4, 201-202.

[36] Germain, A.C. Les *Anciennes Theses de l'Ecole de Médecine de Montpellier*, Memoires de l'Academie des Sciences et des Lettres de Montpellier, 1886, le serie, 7.

[37] Dulieu, 3, (2), 1027-1138.

[38] von Haller, A. *Bibliotheca Chirurgica*, vols 1 & 2. Berne, E Haller & Basilea, and J Schweighauser, 1774, 1, 302.

[39] Dulieu, 3, (1), 530.

[40] Dulieu, 3, (1), 26.

[41] Dulieu, 3, (2), 791-792.

[42] Dulieu, 3, (1), 519.

[43] Vogli, G.G. *Tavole cronologische degli uomini illustri per lettere, e impieghi nudriti dall'Universita di Bologna*, Bologna: Clemente Maria Sassi, 1726.

[44] Astruc, 256.

[45] 1637 not 1638 as stated in the DNB, Dulieu, 3, (1), 798-799.

[46] Dulieu, 3, (2), 989.

[47] *Scharpii G. Institutionum Medicarum pars prima a Claudio Filio in Lucem Edita, Bononiae, apud Jacobum Montium*, 1638.

[48] National Library of Medicine, Bethesda and the Library of the New York Academy of Medicine.

[49] Astruc, 257-258.

[50] Rioux, 25-30.

[51] *Dictionary of National Biography*, 17, 900-901.

[52] Michelet, J. *Histoire de France au dix-septieme Siècle*, reproduced in Oeuvres Completes de Michelet, Paris: Flammarion, 1982, 9, 256-277.

[53] Vic C de et Vaissete HG del. *Histoire generale de Languedoc*, Paris: Jacques Vincent, 1745, 5, 577.

[54] Vic and Vaissete, 538-541.

[55] French names were Les Crinons, Masclous, and Masquelons. Cases in poor children in London were described by Crocker R. Lancet, 1 (1884), 70-71.

[56] Vic and Vaissete, 577.

[57] Henri, Duc de Rohan-Gie, 1579-1638, a favorite of Henry IV, became a Hugenot leader after the assassination of the King.

[58] Dulieu, 3, (2), 786.

[59] The anatomy theatre in Montpellier, built by Rondelet in 1556, was the first in France.

[60] Dulieu, 3, (2), 790.

[61] Dulieu, 3, (2), 799.

The Browne Family at Upton by Chester

The most famous of the Brownes of Upton is Sir Thomas Browne (1605-1682) – physician, scientist, master of literary style, and author of *Religio Medici*. Thomas was born in London, and, after Winchester College, and the Universities of Oxford, Montpellier, Padua, and Leiden, settled in medical practice in Norwich. But his father came from Upton where the family had been settled for many generations.

Upton by Chester and St Mary on the Hill

Upton is nearly two miles north of Chester yet was within the parish of St Mary on the Hill, a Norman church by the Castle and the old Dee Bridge (Figure 2.1).[1] In 1093, the Manor of Upton, belonging to the Earls of Chester, was given to the Abbey of Werburgh, and, at the dissolution of this abbey in 1541, passed to the

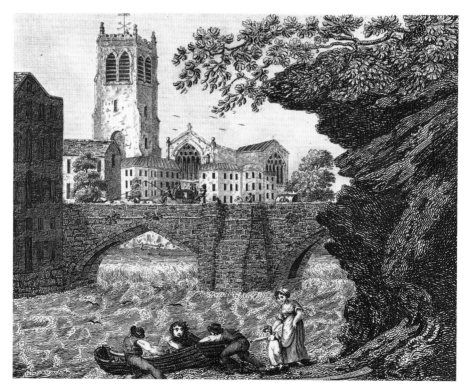

Figure 2.1 An engraving of the Dee and the old Dee bridge and, on rising ground behind them the church of St Mary on the Hill. Altough the image is dated 1798, the engraving was prepared for and reproduced in J Hanshall's History of the County Palatine in Chester in 1817-23.

Episcopal See founded by Henry VIII.[2] In 1553, the Dean and Chapter of the Cathedral granted lands in Upton to Sir Richard Cotton: on his death in 1556, these passed to his son George, who sold the manor to Richard Spencer. It was leased to William Smith in 1576, and, from 1579-80, the Brownes and Brocks were the main fee farmers.[3]

The Church of St. Mary on the Hill stands on high ground overlooking the river Dee, and, built in the early twelfth century by the Earls of Chester, ranked after St Werburg and St John's as one the three great churches of Chester. The parish included Gloverstone within Chester, but extended beyond into five further townships, one of which was Upton.[4] St Mary without the Walls was built and consecrated in 1887 to serve the growing population of Handbridge south of the Dee. In 1972 the old church closed for worship and, being purchased by the County Council in 1975, became a centre for exhibitions and other educational activities.

The Browne Families at Upton and Hoole

An inscribed board – dated 1624 – with a detailed account of the Browne family was mounted on the North wall of St. Mary's by Elizabeth Browne, in memory of her son, Richard Browne, who died in that year.[5] In the early sixteenth century, a Thomas Browne married an Alice White, possibly of Sutton, and this Thomas Browne was the great, great grandfather of Sir Thomas Browne.[6] His son Richard married Katherine Harvey and in 1572 the couple were living in Upton – a prosperous family, bearing arms. A son, Thomas, was born to Richard and Katherine in 1540, and this Thomas Browne (grandfather of Sir Thomas) married Elizabeth, daughter of Henry Birkenhead, Clerk of the Greencloth to Queen Elizabeth. Thomas Browne was a churchwarden at St Mary on the Hill from 1575 to 1576, his partner being Robert Brerewood from another prominent Chester family. Thomas died in 1578 and his will, dated August 18th, 1578, was proved on November 3rd, 1578, when the family home was at Hoole, near Upton.[7] His widow, Elizabeth, died on April 3rd, 1602, and is buried in St Peter's, Chester.[8] (Figure 2.2)Thomas and Katherine had a large family of which the ten names of Henry, Richard, Thomas, Jane, Anne, Edward, William, Ferdinando, Hugh, and Francis are recorded.[9]

Brownes at King's School Chester

This school, founded by Henry VIII in 1541, replaced that of the Monastery of St Werburg. A manuscript register of foundation scholars exists, but may be incomplete and omits pupils other than scholars.[10] In 1547, the first year of record, nine scholars were admitted, and generally the numbers in any year were less than 10, though in some years intake was larger. In 1582, twenty-one scholars were admitted, among them Edward and Ralph Browne. Edward was probably the

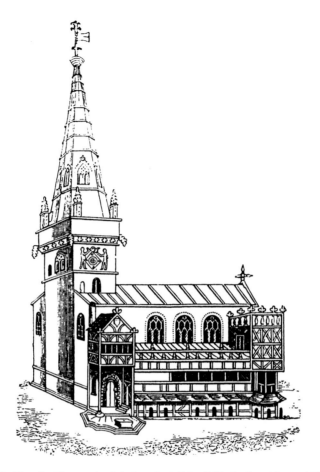

Figure 2.2 St Peter's Church, Chester, burial place in 1602 of Elizabeth, widow of Thomas Browne. This sketch, which appeared in Ormerod's History, reproduces a drawing made by Randle Holmes in the mid seventeenth century. It shows both the old spire, taken down in the late eighteenth century, and the corporation's timber-framed Pentice building which was attached to the south wall of the church.

son of Thomas and Elizabeth and the uncle of Sir Thomas Browne: he was important in the childhood of Browne, when his father died.[11]

Brownes at Brasenose College, Oxford

Henry Browne died in Oxford c.1580, at about the age of 19 years. The second son, Richard Browne, uncle of Sir Thomas Browne, became heir to the family estates, and matriculated at Brasenose on July 4th, 1579, at the age of 17 years. He was a student at Inner Temple in 1583, when his address was at Hoole, Cheshire. In 1587-8, he sold land called the Acres in Upton and Wervin to Henry Birkenhead, and in 1595-6 he sold land called Great Acres to Will Aldersey. Richard Browne died in 1624, and is buried in St Werburgh's, Chester.

Brasenose was the Oxford college of choice for many Chester families. Other Brownes there were Francis Browne, matriculating in 1675 and Benjamin Browne,

within 14 days, there enter a bond with the Chamberlain, and, within a further three months, produce, on pain of imprisonment, an inventory of money, debts, indebtedness, business goods, and personal property.[17] There were other complex requirements, and – pertinent here – the widow was not to remarry before the inventory had been approved by the Common Serjeant.[18] The Court supervised the financial affairs of an orphan until his majority, or for a girl, her marriage or majority. When other evidence is absent, the proceedings of this court may be the sole record of notable events in the childhood of the orphan.

On 9 December, Anne appeared before Cornelius Fish, the Chamberlain of the City of London, with Francis Britridge, a merchant-tailor and her half brother, but without Edward, the other executor. They were bound, in the sum of £2,000, to

> …bring and exhibite into this Court a true and perfect inventory in writing upon her oth therein conteyning all and singuler the goodes chattelles rightes and credittes plate jewelles ready money and debtes which were the said Thomas Brownes' at the tyme of his death.

They were admonished not to 'eloigne and convey the same or any part thereof' out of the 'freedome and liberties' of the City.[19] The inventory was prepared and produced on 10 March 1614. The Common Serjeant entered the total as £5,667 1/2d. The deceased was said to owe £11,209 4s 1d on the day of his death, whilst he was owed, as 'doubtful & desperate debts', £11,514 11s 9d.[20] It was concluded that these figures provided nothing for the widow and orphans. Valuations of the stock of a merchant would be approximate and, whilst outgoing debts would be properly paid out of the estate, it was uncertain how much might be received from what was owed.

Before July 1614, Anne had married Sir Thomas Dutton, and soon evidence of dissent between the two executors appears in the records. The members of the two families, but especially Edward, viewed with alarm the behaviour of Anne and her new husband. On 5 July, the Court of Aldermen appointed Alderman Rotheram, Alderman Bennet the younger, and the Common Serjeant to:

> …examyne and consider the state of Thomas Browne mercer deceased for the setling thereof to the good and benefitt of his orphans and shall examyne the receiptes and disbursements had and made of the said estate since the decease of the said Thomas Browne and shall conferre and deale with Sir Thomas Dutton knight who hath lately married the late wief and executrix of the said Thomas Browne and with Mr Paule Garraway Mr Edward Browne and Mr Frauncis Britteridge who are of neerest blood and aliance to the said orphans… .[21]

The conclusion of 10 March, that Thomas Browne died with a negligible net estate after the counting of debts, was questioned. The two Aldermen and the Common Serjeant were instructed to 'call before them the servantes of the said Thomas Browne deceased for the better effecting & expediting of the said business

...'; this request indicating enquiry into the financial details of the estate. The developing quarrel between Dutton and Edward Browne was addressed: 'And the said Committee shall likewise heare and end all matters in Controversie between the said Sir Thomas Dutton and the said Edward Browne...'. If the 'Controversie' could not be resolved the 'Lord Maior' was to be 'elected umpier in the said cause...'[22]

The majesty and powers of the Court had the desired effect, the quarrel abated and new figures were calculated. On 14 July, Sir Thomas Middleton, the Lord Mayor, presided over the Court which discovered several facts.[23] It was agreed that Anne Browne and Edward Browne had both been appointed executors but that Anne alone had proved the will and had taken upon herself its execution and the exhibition of an inventory. The figures given for the estate were as before, saving the incorporation of funeral and other charges of £250. The amount standing to the credit of the estate was calculated as £5,722 7s 7½d. Amongst the debts some were thought, by friends and servants, 'very desperate & much of the rest doubtfull', giving a realistic estimate of £3,222 7s 7d 'or theraboutes'. Anne's conduct in the past few months were criticised:

> ...the said Anne the executrix sithence the decease of her said husband hath altered the propertie of as many of the debtes owing... and taken them in her owne name as amounteth to the summe of ml vCli [£1,500].

It was thought that:

> ...it is likely and very much to be feared that unlesse somme speedy Course be taken for setling therof that very great losse will fall to the five orphans... .[24]

The Court of Aldermen was distrustful of Dutton and of his profession as a soldier:

> ...for that shee is now lately married to Sir Thomas Dutton knight, who although he be a very worthy gent yet it may be feared that he being a Marshall man may live beyond the seas, or in the countrey, and soe out of the jurisdiccion and power of this Court.[25]

The worthy burghers were alarmed by this soldier knight and knew his reputation for choleric swordsmanship, for he had, in a notorious duel, killed his commanding officer. The Court settled with the pair for a sum calculated to end their influence in the estate:

> ...after many offers and profers made it is demaunded and stood upon by the said Sir Thomas Dutton and Dame Anne his wief & either of them that for the relinquishment of the executorshipp or at the least of any further medling or dealing hereafter as Executrix there may be allowed unto them out of the estate of the said Testator or the summe of... .[26]

Sir Thomas and Anne were to be bought off with £1,000, of which £500 was immediately payable and £500 in six months. The Court ruefully calculated

£1,542 10s 1d as the price of being rid of the couple. Notwithstanding, on 4 August, Dutton and Anne returned to the Court with a claim that wares had been sold for £38 10s less than the sum at which they were valued, and giving further details of Anne's living expenses, including her lying in expenses, as Ellen had now been born.[27]

On 27 August the Court appointed Francis Brittridge and Christopher Rotheram to represent the Duttons, who '...shall noe further intermeddle as executores and the said Edward Browne alone shall administer...'.[28] On 8 September, Edward certified that he owed £2,000 to the Chamberlain for the orphans, which account he had paid on 15 November.[29] This judgement was satisfactory, as there are no more entries in the records of the Corporation of London relating to these orphans for eight years, when entries record the majority of each of the five children.

Thomas Browne signed his own satisfaction on 19 November 1629, and Christopher Rotheram testified that he was over 21.[30] Browne was then 24 and that year had proceeded to a MA at Oxford. His address on admission to Winchester College, both in August 1616 and in the Election Roll of August 1622 was St Michael le Cheape, Middlesex (correctly St Michael le Querne, Cheapside).[31] This was also his address on matriculation at Broadgates Hall in the University of Oxford.[32]

There were four sisters, Anne, Mary, Jane, and Ellen, whose fortunes are sparsely documented and, because of the Great Fire, their records of baptism in the registers of St Michael le Querne have been lost. Anne was the first born. She married John Palmer on 30 December 1628, in the church of St Martin Pomeroy, Ironmonger Lane.[33] The Court of Aldermen records her attendance on 21 April 1629. The Repertory entry reads:

> ...Item John Palmer Citizen and Grocer of London and Anne his wife one of the daughters and late orphans of Thomas Browne late Citizen and Mercer of London deceased here present doe acknowledge themselves fully satisfied and paid of all such mony as groweth due unto them... And therof they doe discharge this Court and the said Recognitors bound for the same.[34]

Well done, Edward Browne. He had supported his niece, and found her a husband from the Grocers' Company. It is likely that Anne lived in London for many of the 14 years from her mother's second marriage to her own marriage.

Mary was the second daughter and the second to marry, on 30 September 1630, at St Michael, Paternoster Royal.[35] The bridegroom was Nevill Craddock of Clifford's Inn. The Court of Orphans was involved, in that, before the marriage, Nevill Craddock had entered into a bond for £250 that '...in consideracion of the porcion of the said Mary which she should received with her in marriage...', he agreed to leave her £200 for her own use.[36] On 19 April 1631 Mary signed a satisfaction that she had received payment of her final portion.[37] Neville Craddock died in 1653, and his will was proved in June of that year. Dr Browne and his wife and his children were on good terms with the Craddock family and at least twelve letters mention news and visits between Norwich and London.[38]

Jane, the third sister, probably went with Ellen and her mother to Ireland, or, at least, spent some time there. She married Thomas Price of Drumlaham in County Cavan, Ireland in 1632 or 1633. The Court required a satisfaction on her behalf, and this was signed by Neville Craddock, Jane's brother in law, on 4 February 1634.[39] Jane made an excellent match, since Price proceeded to an illustrious career in the church in Ireland.[40] Born of a Welsh family in London, he attended Trinity College, Dublin, where he gained his BA in 1623 and was elected a Fellow in 1626. He proceeded to a MA in 1628. Ordained by Bishop Bedell, he became successively Archdeacon of Kilmore in 1638, Bishop of Kildare in 1660, and Archbishop of Cashel in 1667.[41] He died in Cashel in 1685. His will suggests that Jane died before him.[42] There is no mention of children. Browne remained in touch and on friendly terms with his sister Jane and her husband, but his mother is never mentioned. In a letter to his son Edward dated 1682 he asks to be remembered to the Archbishop of Cashel.[43]

Ellen, the youngest and born soon after the death of her father in 1613, lived with her mother in Ireland, and there are few records of her in England. On 23 April 1639 she signed a satisfaction that she had received her portion of the will and Edward Browne deposed that she was now over twenty one.[44] She was then aged 26 years and probably was rarely in London.

None of the depositions concerning the five children mention Sir Thomas and Lady Dutton, which omission from the many statements is significant, although the Court had excluded the couple from direct involved in the estate.

Browne's mother was born Anne Garraway, one of four children of Paul Garraway, who married Alice Britridge, born Page.[45] Paul Garraway died in April 1620 and Philip Garraway, of Acton, Middlesex, the eldest son, became the executor of his father's estate. Philip died in 1625, and his will came to probate in April 1625.

The main inheritor was Roger Britridge, the half brother of Philip, but a ring worth five pounds was left to Lady Dutton, the sister of Philip and the mother of Browne. Philip Garraway remained in touch with his sister and her new family, and small legacies remembered her recent children, Thomas and William Dutton.

Browne recollected his maternal grandfather in Sussex in a letter to his son, Edward, dated 9 January 1681 (old style), which mentioned a visit: '...when I was very yong & I thinck butt in coates, my mother carryed mee to my Grandfather Garrawayes howse in Lewys. I retaine only in my mind the idea of some roomes of the howse and of the church...'.[46] This is the sole mention of his mother in Browne's large surviving correspondence, and it is the only link between Lewes, Sussex, and Anne, who probably came from Acton, Middlesex.

When Anne Browne remarried, she could not have chosen, from English suitors, a more dissimilar second husband. She had buried a pious, industrious London merchant; she married Sir Thomas Dutton, a swashbuckling soldier of an illustrious Cheshire family. It is probable that Anne had known Thomas Dutton for some time and possibly before her marriage to Thomas Browne. The Garraway family had connections with Acton, Middlesex, the home of her brother Philip. Thomas Dutton, although from a Cheshire family, was born in Isleworth, Middlesex, and later, the married couple lived in his house. Acton is to the north-east of Isleworth, both villages being adjacent on the north bank of the river Thames. There may be another link with the Dutton family in that a sister of Thomas Browne – the father of Sir Thomas Browne – and also called Anne Browne, married John Dutton, of Guilden, Sutton, for her second husband.

The Great Rebellion in Ireland began in 1641 and for Anne, now a widow and living with Ellen, times were perilous. The plantation had confiscated the lands of the Farrell family and the Duttons living on these or nearby estates were a target for revenge. Oliver Boy Fitzgerald of Longford 'hanged 16 English there & stript the Lady Dutton of all her goods and clothes...'. 'Lady Ann Dutton & her daughter Mrs. Elinor Browne; her man, her mayde ...were threatened to be put to death...' deposed John Stibbs of Longford. The reference to 'Mrs Elinor Browne' is not reliable evidence that Elinor had married. A 'Cabinet Council' instructed Captain Fergus Farell to execute the Dutton family but they were saved by the prompt action of Lady Newcommen, who alerted Sir James Dillon. Sir James rescued them into his own house and conveyed them safely to the garrison in Athlone.[47] The subsequent fate of Lady Dutton and Ellen is unknown. Possibly they came to England but probably they remained in Ireland on what remained of their estate. Poor Anne, again a widow, had exchanged her London family and friends for a turbulent life with a soldier with ambitions in Ireland.

The history of the Duttons of Dutton places Sir Thomas as the black sheep of the family.[48] Thomas Dutton was born in 1575 in Isleworth, Middlesex, the son of John Dutton. He was knighted in 1603 amongst the plethora of creations of King James I.[49] He was admitted to Gray's Inn in 1605, but turned to the Army, serving in the Low Countries, and in Ireland, where, in 1610, he was appointed Scoutmaster-General. Before and after his marriage to Anne in 1614 – his second marriage – he was chiefly engaged in Ireland, where, in 1619, he was granted 2,000 acres in the Longford Plantation. Dutton was known to James I, Charles I, and Charles II, and was usually in their favour, except for a period after the fatal duel.[50] State documents abound with mention of this reckless soldier, usually recording the soliciting of persons in high places for money or advantage.[51] Dutton lived in self-created penury, periodically improved by financial windfalls, such as his marriage to the widow, Anne Browne. His life ended in 1634, typically after injuries sustained in a London brawl 'amongst Low-Country friends ...'.[52]

Browne's firstborn was named Edward, not Thomas, Browne's own name and that of his father. But Browne had married Dorothy Mileham, whose father was Edward and this was their first consideration. By an appropriate coincidence, his uncle, Edward Browne was also remembered, a guardian to whom Browne must have been grateful throughout his career, founded on attendance at a good school and university, and extensive European travel, all made possible by the wise guardianship of Edward, who deserves further mention. Migrating to London from Chester, he became a grocer, being apprenticed to Martin Archedale in 1587.[53] He obtained his freedom in 1594, and was taken into livery in 1604.[54] He retired in 1620, and was alive in 1639, when he certified that Ellen Browne was over twenty one.[55]

The events narrated above, chiefly drawn from the records of the Court of Aldermen, invite speculation on Browne's affinity for his parents and stepfather. Browne's father, an industrious merchant, died in 1613, when Browne was eight years old. His sudden illness and death caused his children great distress, although the will made good provision for the widow and children. His wife, although joint executor with Edward Browne, proved the will alone. This prompted the Court to require Anne, and her half brother Francis, to bring certain information, which proved unacceptable, the more so as Anne had remarried and there was 'controversie' between her new husband and Edward, the other executor. Conferences between Anne, Anne's father, Edward, Francis, and Dutton, decided on an arrangement whereby Anne and Dutton had some £1,500 from the estate provided that they cease to '...meddle any further in the execution...'. The Court considered this bargain 'excessive' but nevertheless instructed Edward to prove the will [again] and to execute the estate alone. The character of Dutton, in debt for most of his life, and marrying Anne for her money is transparently clear. However, Browne's mother appears in a scarcely better light, and seems irresponsible towards the three elder children.

Browne was on good terms with two of his sisters. No letters survive to or from Anne and John Palmer but several show his friendship with both Mary and Jane, and with their families. Ellen was in Ireland during Browne's early years of travel, which explains why there is no record of any exchange of letters or news. Browne seems not to have corresponded with his mother – at least no correspondence has survived – but his feelings towards her can be conjectured. Orphaned at eight, at boarding school for eight years from the age of ten, and subsequently away in Oxford and in Europe, he was seldom in the company of his mother after early childhood. He must later have pondered on his mother's rash remarriage, and the character of his stepfather, Dutton, who was briefly his companion on a tour of Ireland.

The will of Sir Thomas Dutton, who died in 1634, was lost by fire in the troubles of Dublin in 1922, but it mentioned his wife Anne, his heir Charles, and sons William and Thomas.[56] After Dutton's death, where Browne's mother lived, and where she died, are not recorded, and her fate seems to have been unknown to Browne. A powerful influence on the life and work of Browne was the death of his father. Soon after, his contact with his mother became infrequent, to the extent of complete separation. Browne was intensely religious and knew the words of Psalm 27 '…When my father and my mother forsake me, then the Lord will take me up…'.

ACKNOWLEDGEMENTS

I am grateful for facilities in the Bodleian Library, Oxford, and in the Guildhall Library, London; and, for the use of records, to the Worshipful Companies of Mercers and Grocers, to Winchester College, and to Trinity College, Dublin. I am especially indebted to the Corportion of London Record Office for photocopies of the records of the Court of Orphans, which form the basis of the research reported here.

NOTES AND REFERENCES

1 Whitlock B.W, 'The Orphange Accounts of John Donne, Ironmonger', *Guildhall Miscellany*, 1 (1955), 22-29.

2 [John Hase ?] *Posthumous Works of the learned Sir Thomas Browne* (1712), xxxvi. Whether Hase, or the publisher, J. Payne was the author of the life is uncertain.

3 *Life* by Samuel Johnson, included in *Christian Morals by Sir Thomas Browne of Norwich, M.D.* 1756, ii and iii.

4 Williams C, 'The Will of Thomas Browne, Mercer, Cheapside, London', *Proceedings of the Norfolk and Norwich Archaeological Society*, 16 (1905-7), 132-146.

5 Osler W, 'An Address on Sir Thomas Browne', *British Medical Journal*, 2 (1905), 993-998.

6 Gosse E, *Sir Thomas Browne*. New York: Macmillan Co, 1905. Reprinted Westport, Connecticut: Greenwood Press, 1970.

7 Finch J.S, *Sir Thomas Browne: A Doctor's Life of Science and Faith*. New York: Henry Schuman, 1950, 29.

8 Huntley F.L, *Sir Thomas Browne: A Biographical and Critical Study* Ann Arbor, USA: University of Michigan Press, 1968, 6.

9 Bennett J, *Sir Thomas Browne: A Man of Achievement in Literature*. Cambridge: Cambridge University Press, 1962, 2-5.

10 Endicott N.J, 'Sir Thomas Browne as "Orphan", with some account of his Stepfather, Sir Thomas Dutton', *University of Toronto Quarterly*, 30 (1961), 180-210.

11 Mercers' Company, *Names of All Freemen, 1594*. There is also a typescript list, where the entry appears in Vol A-C, 52.

12 Mercers' Company, *Acts of Court, 1595-1629, f. 57v.*

13 ibid, *f. 115.*

14 ibid, *ff. 126 and 129v.*

[15] The will is: 1613 Browne, Thomas, *Probate Act Book, St Michael le Querne, 123 Capell*. The original is held by the Public Record Office.

[16] Carlton C.H, 'The Administration of London's Court of Orphans', *Guildhall Miscellany*, 4 (1971), 27.

[17] Carlton C.H, *The Court of Orphans*. Leicester: 1974.

[18] Carlton, 'Administration of London's Court of Orphans', 22-35.

[19] Corporation of London Records Office (CLRO), *Repertory (Rep) 31 (2), f. 224v*.

[20] CLRO, *Orphanage, Common Serjeant's Book, 1, f. 417v*.

[21] CLRO, *Rep. 31 (2), f. 356*.

[22] ibid.

[23] ibid, ff. *372v-375*.

[24] ibid.

[25] ibid.

[26] ibid.

[27] ibid, *ff. 386v-387*.

[28] ibid, *ff. 389v-390*.

[29] ibid, *ff. 395v-396 and f. 8*.

[30] CLRO, *Rep. 44, ff. 20v-21*.

[31] Winchester College: Register of Scholars *vol. 1 f. 111* and Muniment Room, *Election Roll for 1622*

[32] Archives of the University of Oxford. *Registrum Matriculatum 1615-1647, PP2, f. 267*, under *Aula Lateportensis*.

[33] Guildhall Library *(GL), MS. 4392*.

[34] CLRO, *Rep.43, f. 147*.

[35] GL. *MS. 5142*.

[36] CLRO, *Orphans Recognizances 5, f. 58v*.

[37] CLRO, *Rep. 45, ff, 245v-246*.

[38] Keynes G, (ed.), *The Works of Sir Thomas Browne* London 1928-1931, Faber and Gwyer, becoming Faber and Faber, vi, 49, 100, 123, 132, 140, 180, 188, 200, 213, 235, and 255.

[39] CLRO, *Letter Book HH, ff. 124-124v*, and *Rep. 48, ff. 95-95v*.

[40] *Dictionary of National Biography*, xvi 1909, 340.

[41] Archbishop Price is important because of his attempts to use the Irish language in the established church in Ireland.

[42] Vicars A.E, *Index to the Prerogative Wills of Ireland*, (1897), 81 and 386. The will has not survived; for details see references to Price in the DNB.

[43] Keynes, vi, 265.

[44] CLRO, *Letter Book HH, f. 124*, and *Rep. 53, ff. 166v-167*.

[45] Tildesley M.L, 'Sir Thomas Browne: His Skull, Portraits, and Ancestry', *Biometrika*, 15 (1923), 55-56.

[46] Keynes, vi, 233-234. The only mention in 232 letters.

[47] Trinity College, Dublin, *MSS, 1641 depositions Longford, 134 and 204*, and *MS 830, 1641 depositions, Rescommon, 2*.

[48] I am indebted for details of Dutton to Dr. N. J. Endicott. See Endicott N.J, 'Sir Thomas

Insignes.[16] Riverius is one of the five authorities on diseases "...which are of singular benefit". wrote Browne to his protégé Henry Power.[17]

In 1630, Lazarre Rivière treated the King, whose progress through southern France paused at Lyon. On October 2nd his life was saved by the spontaneous rupture of a peri-anal abscess, "ignores des docteurs" who had bled their patient into a state of anaemia.[18] Rivière has the reputation of introducing to Montpellier the type of chemical medicaments proposed by Paracelsus, one notable example being antimony, in the use of which the medical schools of Montpellier and Paris were opposed. Innovative Montpellier explored chemical remedies whilst conservative Paris preferred Galenicals. The academic conflict came to be known as *La guerre de l'antimoine*.[19] Passions ran high between the two ancient medical schools and Gui Patin, Professor of Medicine in Paris, was critical of the writings of Rivière, and all Montpellier physicians. But history esteems Riviere as one of the first physicians in France and one who championed the work of Harvey.

Martin Richer de Beleval (1599-1664) (Figure 4.2) was Dean of the Medical School and Professor of Anatomy, and the nephew of Pierre Richer de Belleval (1564-1632), who created the celebrated Jardin des Plantes in Montpellier for Henri IV. Pierre appointed his nephew to the chairs of Anatomy and Botany, and to the directorship of the botanical garden. Browne would have been taught anatomy and botany by Martin, have known of Pierre, and would have visited the great botanical garden, then being replanted following its destruction in the siege of Montpellier in 1622. Browne's interest in botany and horticulture arose in Montpellier.

Francois Ranchin (1560-1641), born and educated in Montpellier, became Professor in 1605, and Chancellor in 1612. He was known as a senior figure in the University, and as an administrator, being active in the reconstruction of Montpellier after the destruction of the city in 1622, and in the rebuilding of the anatomy theatre of Guillaume Rondelet.[20] Ranchin's medical and administrative abilities were tested in the terrible outbreak of plague in 1629-1630, during which, as Mayor of Montpellier, he showed great courage and energy in rallying the city to such measures of containing the outbreak as were possible, which events immediately preceded Browne's arrival. Browne's library contained Ranchin's *Opuscula Medica*, 1627, and *De Morbis Ante Partum*, 1645.[21]

Browne's Life in Montpellier

Delaunay describes the medical curriculum in seventeenth-century Montpellier.[22] Students lodged where they could afford, sometimes in return for services. Later, Browne wrote to his son, Tom, in France "...live with an Apothecairie...", and it is likely that Browne himself lodged with an apothecary.[23] The students were required to dine together at midday. Instruction was given in the primitive medical school whose buildings have been researched by Bonnet.[24] Today the site is occupied by the Department of Pharmacy flanked by the Rue du Calvaire and the Rue Ecole de Pharmacie. The nearby church of Notre Dame des Tables, used for tuition by the medical school, was destroyed in the French Revolution, and only its ruins and crypt remain. How Browne found these structures in 1630 is uncertain as the city was being rebuilt following the destruction of 1622. Medical students were frequently intemperate and disorderly, and the summer hot, as Browne remembered when he bade "Honest Tom" to "...live soberly and temperately, the heat of that place will otherways mischief you".[25]

Browne's tolerance of the religions of others, and his acceptance of practices other than his own, began in Montpellier, as he recollected in *Religio Medici* "Whilst, therefore, they directed their devotions to Her, I offered mine to God...".[26] Browne was not prejudiced about the food he ate: "I wonder not at the French for their dishes of Frogs, Snails, and Toadstools... but being amongst them... I find they agree with my stomach as well as theirs".[27] Browne's was intrigued by the metamorphosis of the silkworm: "Those strange and mystical transmigrations that I have observed in Silk-worms, turned my Philosophy into Divinity".[28]

Montpellier and Languedoc in the Religious Wars

France, ruled by Louis XIII and Cardinal Richelieu, was riven by the struggles between Catholics and Protestants. Montpellier, Languedoc and Southern France were greatly disturbed in these local conflicts, which were followed by famine and outbreaks of plague. The Hugenots were a minority group, scarce in the North but numerous in the South. Protestants were a majority in Montpellier and controlled the town, which Louis sieged in 1622, devastating the town and destroying most of its buildings before its surrender and the peace of Montpellier signed in October 1622. By 1629, England and France were at peace, but meanwhile Richelieu and the King savagely subdued the south of France. The devastation from the royal army brought the plague, which, in Montpellier, began at the end of July 1629, and, by November, two thousand inhabitants had died.[29] The epidemic lessened in December and had ceased by February 1630, by which time the towns of Pui, Carcassone, Montauban, and Toulouse were affected.

Browne came to a still stricken city, and the matriculation entry of seven persons in 1629 compared with 33 in 1630 indicates the reduced activity of the University of Montpellier in 1629. Also significant was the prevalence of Morgellons, an illness now forgotten by the medical profession, but associated with extreme poverty.[30] Browne must have grieved deeply at the suffering that surrounded him. Yet, only thirty four years later his son Edward found the town much altered as is evident in his letter to his father dated October 7th, 1664.

> This place is the most delightfull of all France, being seated upon an hill in sight of the sea; inhabited by a people... the most handsome in the world... I live at an apothecary's house... In the physick garden here, I meet with many things which are neither in England nor Paris.[31]

Padua

Lucentio, in the *Taming of the Shrew* (first performed c. 1596), coming from his native Pisa, acknowledges the superiority of the University of Padua, where in 1602 William Harvey obtained his MD. Padua was the most celebrated medical school in the world and, in the sixteenth century, pupils from England included the founders of the Royal College of Physicians, the most famous being Thomas Linacre.[32] Of the ancient universities of Italy in the thirteenth century, Bologna, Pisa, and Pavia were renowned, and migration from Bologna in 1222 created Padua. From the fourteenth century, Venice supported the nearby University of Padua, which served the most important city in the world. The independence from Rome was an important factor, especially as Padua welcomed Protestants, ignoring a papal decree against non-catholics in Italian universities.

Many famous names catalogue the sustained rise of the school of medicine. Paolo Bagellardi (d. 1492 or 1494) is the father of paediatrics, and the author of the first printed book on diseases of children. Girolamo Fracastoro (1483-1553) – professor of medicine at Padua – introduced epidemiology, and his book *De contagione* proposes a scientific mechanism for the transmission of disease. The speciality of dermatology begins with Girolamo Mercuriale (1530-1606), and occupational medicine with Bernardino Ramazzini (1633-1714). But teaching anatomy brought the most fame to Padua, with three renowned anatomists: Andreas Vesalius (1514-1564), Gabrielle Fallopio (1523-1563), and Fabrizi d'Acquependente (1533-1619). In Padua was built the first anatomy theatre, where thousands of doctors, scientists, and painters observed demonstrations by the professor of anatomy: at about the time of Browne, this was Johannes Vesling (1598-1649), also professor of botany.[33] Vesling, from Minden, had studied the flora of the middle east whilst Consul in Cairo.[34] Browne possessed the 1666 edition of Vesling's *Syntagma Anatomicum*, illustrated by G. Blasio.[35]

Measurement in physiology began in Padua by Santorio Santorio (1561-1636), a friend of Galileo, whose techniques of measurement in physics were applied to biology and medicine,[36] (Figure 4.3).[37] He invented the clinical thermometer, the hygrometer, and a pendulum pulse-clock. Browne may have been taught by Santorio and knew his work, having two of his books.[38] Many years later he wrote on the permeability of the skin to perspiration which:

> Sanctorius first discovered by staticall trialls and experiments, by wayghing men's bodyes at divers times, that the whole masse of effluviums amounted to a greater wayght than what was excluded by seidge and urine.[39]

The exact date of Browne's period in Padua is uncertain but it is likely that he arrived in the autumn of 1632, when the academic year began. Lectures

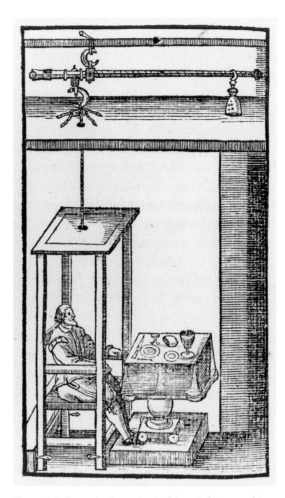

Figure 4.3 Santorio Santorio, in his weighing machine.
From an engraving in *De Statica Medicina*, Leiden, 1642.

continued until the following August, with tuition every weekday except Thursdays. There is no record of Browne in the matriculation book, but we find again the name of Thomas Nott, of London. Browne came to Padua at a period in the thirty years war, when this part of Italy was recovering from devastation, famine, and plague, the main conflict being between Spain and France. France wished to sever the land and river route *via* the Rhine between Spain and its possessions in the low countries, and to this end was fought the War of the Mantuan succession. In 1630 German troops sieged Mantua, destroyed the Venetian army, and sacked the town. Venice was saved by the intervention of a Swedish army, supported by France, but plague reduced the population of Venice by a third and devastated many cities in Northern Italy. The recovery of Venice was limited: its port and trade was declining, and this permanently affected Padua and its university.[40]

Leiden

The University of Leiden, founded in 1575 by William the Silent, swiftly became a leading university, with a famous medical school.[41] The older University of Louvain – founded in 1426 – was reserved for Roman Catholics, but Leiden welcomed Catholics, Protestants, and Jews, a religious tolerance evident in its many settlers and pilgrims: it was the port from which many proceeded to New England. In 1633 – the year of Browne's attendance – the medical school was thronged by students from many countries, attracted by modern medical tuition. The young Dutch Republic, emerging from the domination of Spain, was attaining wealth and power, and its formidable navy harried the sea connection between Spain and the Low Countries.

Browne matriculated on Dec. 3rd and obtained his MD on Dec. 21, 1633, the entry in the Acta stating "...[42] Visus est dignus Thomas Browne, cui supremus in Medicina gradus conferatur, quem illi tribuit D. Vorstius". His stay in Leiden was probably longer and possibly a year. For his doctorate Browne would have submitted a dissertation called a 'Thesis pro gradu Doctoratus' which he would have defended in the presence of the Praeses and other professors, usually in public. The thesis has not survived, nor is the title known.[43] Theses were in manuscript till 1600, when they became printed.

In 1633 Adrian van Valkenburg was the anatomist.[44] Anatomy teaching in Leiden began with Pieter Paaw (1564-1617), who had studied under Fabricius in Padua. Paaw built the anatomy theatre, but was also a botanist and director of the Botanical Garden. Browne describes Paaw as "a famous Professor of Leyden, dissected a Gulo'[wolverine]", and, in commenting how difficult it is to examine the human spinal cord, refers to this being accomplished by Paaw.[45] Adolphus Vorstius (1597-1663) was professor of Botany and presented Browne for his degree.[46] Jan de Wale (1604-1649) was appointed Professor Extraordinary of Medicine in 1633, the year of Browne in Leiden.

Anatomy, botany, and medicine were thriving in Leiden, but other subjects were developing, particularly in the Low Countries. Chemistry was advanced by Van Helmont who, following Paracelsus, in turn, influenced Sylvius (Figure 4.4).[47] Franciscus de le Boe Sylvius (1614-72) was a student in Leiden c. 1634, slightly after Browne, who had two of his books.[48] Proceeding MD at Basel in 1638, Sylvius returned to Leiden and to hostile criticism from de Wale, who was later converted to the methods of Sylvius. Wale's experiments on ligations of the veins and arteries of the living dog were an important confirmation of the work of Harvey, who published *De motu cordis* in 1628.[49]

Conclusion

Browne returned to England with a superb grounding in anatomy, botany, physiology, chemistry, and medical practice, together with a knowledge of several European countries and their languages. His next academic move –

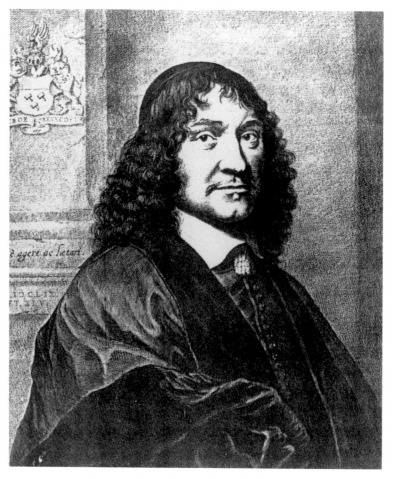

Figure 4.4 Franciscus de le Boe Sylvius.
From a 1659 engraving by Cornelis van Dalen Jr.

essential for his medical practice in Norwich – was to incorporate his Leiden degree into an Oxford DM, which ceremony took place on July 10th 1637, the minimum period of fourteen years having intervened since his matriculation in Oxford (Figure 4.5).[50] During the preceding three years he engaged in some medical practice and wrote Religio Medici, from which his fame endures. Following Browne in Europe, we have traced the pattern of education of many English (and Scots and Irish) physicians, who, having studied abroad, returned to practice, after incorporating an Oxford or Cambridge degree.

ACKNOWLEDGEMENTS

I am grateful to the staff of the Bodleian Library, Oxford, the Britsh Library, and the Public Record Office, and to the archivists of the University of Oxford, Montpellier, Padua and Leiden.

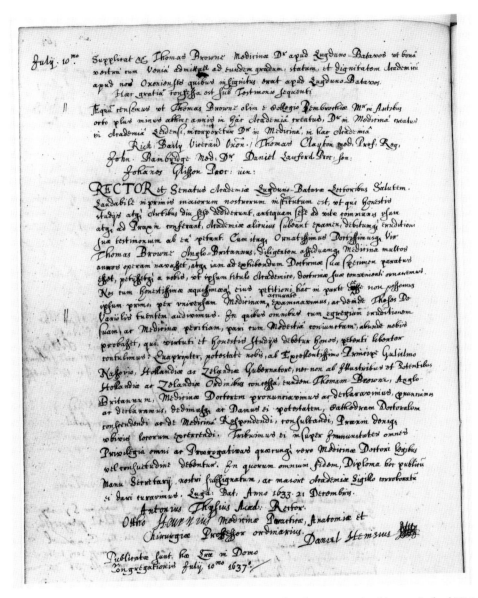

Figure 4.5 Record of the incorporation of Browne's Leiden degree granting him an Oxford DM. (reproduced by permission of the Oxford University Archivist: Incorporation, NEP/ Supra Q, 10 July 1637, f.162v.)

NOTES AND REFERENCES

[1] Browne T. *The Works of Sir Thomas Browne* (henceforth Works). Vols 1-6. Keynes G, ed. London: Faber and Gwyer (becoming Faber and Faber), 1928-31.

[2] Ballard T. Bookseller. *A Catalogue of the Libraries of the Learned Sir Thomas Brown, and Dr Edward Brown, his Son ... Which Will begin to be sold by Auction ... on Monday the 8th day of January, 1710/11 .... at the Rising-Sun in Little Britain.* (Henceforth Catalogue).

[3] The Public Record Office has no record of a passport for Browne, as e.g., was provided on 18 June 1631 for: 'John Kent, George Bates & Robert Brownelowe... Oxford ...to goe over to Lydon in the Lowe Countries ...to better their knowledge of Physicke'. Passes specified towns to be visited and often excluded Rome and Spain.

[4] Hughes J. T. 'The Childhood of Sir Thomas Browne : Evidence from the Court of Orphans', *London Journal*, 23, (1998), 24-29.

[5] Kellett CE. 'Sir Thomas Browne and the disease called the Morgellons'. *Annals of Medical History*, 7, (1935); 467-79.

[6] *Works*, 5, 95-6. In Browne's *Miscellany Tracts*, 8.

[7] *Works*, 1, 50. In *Religio Medici* (henceforth RM), 39.

[8] James Primerose dedicated *Academio Monspeliensis*, 1631 to Thomas Clayton. Browne knew Primerose, who incorporated his Montpellier MD at Oxford in March 1628. Prolific but unsound, Primerose wrote *De Vulgi in Medicina Erroribus* in 1638 (English translation 1651) before Browne's *Pseudodoxia Epidemica*, published in 1646.

[9] *Works*, 6, 7. Letter from Browne to Tom, dated November 1, 1661.

[10] Guthrie D. *A History of Medicine*. London: Thomas Nelson, 1945, 113.

[11] The modern extensive account is Dulieu L. *La Médecine à Montpellier*. Vols 1-4, Avignon: Les Presses Universelles, 1975-90, the relevant volume being Tome 3, L'Epoque Classique. Shorter is Dulieu L. *La Médecine a Montpellier du XII au XX siècle*. Paris: Hervas, 1990; and Bonnet H. *La Faculté de Médecine de Montpellier*. Montpellier: Sauramps Medical, 1992. Older references are in *Rashdall's Universities of Europe in the Middle Ages. Vols 1-3*, Powicke FM and Emden AB eds. Oxford : Clarendon Press, 1936, 2, 116-139.

[12] Montpellier suffered a serious epidemic of plague in 1629.

[13] Thomas Nott subsequently obtained a medical degree at Padua, October 27th, 1632.

[14] Astruc J. *Mémoires pour servir a l'Histoire de la Faculté de Medēcine de Montpellier*. Paris: P.-G. Cavelier Libraire, 1767.

[15] George Scharpe was a clever, but quarrelsome, and intemperate Scotsman, who in 1634, moved to Bologna, where he died in 1638. *Dictionary of National Biography*. London: Smith, Elder & Co., 1908: vol. 17, 900-1.

[16] *Catalogue*, p.24, nos. 53 and 54, and p.57, no.19.

[17] *Works*, 6, 278. Letter to Dr Henry Power, 1646.

[18] Michelet J. *Histoire de France au Dix-Septième Siècle*. Paris: 1857. Vol 9 of *Oeuvres Completes*: Paris, 1990, p.275.

[19] Packard FR. *Guy Patin and the Medical Profession in Paris in the XVIIth Century*. New York: Hoeber, 1924, Reprint New York: Kelley, 1970, 198-238.

[20] The anatomy theatre in Montpellier, built by Rondelet in 1556, was the first in France.

21 *Catalogue*, p.21, no.51, and p.25, 94

22 Delaunay P. La Vie Médicale aux XVIe, XVIIe, et XVIIIe Siècles. Paris : Editions Hippocrate, 1935.

23 *Works*, 6, 7. Letter to Tom, March 10th, 1660-1.

24 Bonnet, 130-1.

25 *Works*, 6, 8. Letter to Tom, March 10th, 1660-1.

26 *Works*, 1, 7. RM, 1, 3.

27 *Works*, 1, 72. RM, 2, 1.

28 *Works*, 1, 50. RM, 1, 39.

29 Vic C de et Vaissete HG deL. Histoire Générale de Languedoc, Volume 5, Paris : Jacques Vincent, 1745, p.577.

30 French names were Les Crinons, Masclous, and Masquelons. Cases in poor children of London were described by Crocker R. *Lancet*, 1884, 1, 704.

31 MS Sloane, 1868. Letters to Browne are reproduced in *Sir Thomas Browne's Works*, Wilkin S, ed. London: William Pickering , 1836, 1, 70-1.

32 Castiglioni A. 'The Medical School at Padua and the Renaissance of Medicine'. *Annals of Medical History*, (N.S.) 7 (1935), 214-27. For early references see Rashdall, 2, 9-21.

33 Tomasini JP. *Gymnasium Patavini. Utini* : Nicola Schiratti, 1654.

34 *Biografia Universale*. Venezia : Presso Gio Batista Missiaglia, 1830, Vol 59, pp. 452-3.

35 *Catalogue*, p.19, no.2.

36 Castiglioni A. 'The Life and Work of Sanctorius', *Medical Life*, 38 (1931), 729-86.

37 The figure is reproduced from Sanctorii S. *De Statica Medicina*. Leiden : David Lopes de Haro, 1642, facing p.1.

38 *Catalogue*, p.21, nos.53 and 54.

39 MS Sloane 1848. In *Miscellaneous Writings*, f.17. Reproduced in Works, 5, 304.

40 Lane FC. Venice : *A Maritime Republic*. Baltimore and London : Johns Hopkins University Press, 1973, 400.

41 Lusingh Scheurleer ThH and Posthumus Meyjes GHM. *Leiden University in the Seventeenth* Century. Leiden: Universitaire Pers Leiden/EJ Brill, 1975.

42 Innes Smith RW. *English-Speaking Students of Medicine at the University of Leyden*. Edinburgh and London: Oliver and Boyd, 1932, 34.

43 The Bodleian and British libraries and those of the British Medical Association and Royal Society of Medicine have some seventeenth century Leyden theses but not that of Browne.

44 *Nieuw Nederlandsch Biographisch Woordenboek*. Leiden: , 1911-37, Vol.4, 1357.

45 *Works*, 6, 86 and 98. Letters to Edward Browne, March 7, 1676-1677 and July 6 1678.

46 Veendorp H. and Baas Becking LGM. *Hortus Academicus Lugduno-Batavus 1587-937*. Harlem: 1938, 68-75.

47 Spronsen JW van. 'The Rise of Chemistry as an Independent Science'. In Lunsingh Scheurleer, 329-43.

48 *Catalogue*, p.27, nos. 41 and 42.

49 Lindeboom GA. 'Dog and Frog: Physiological experiments at Leiden during the 17th century'. In Lungsingh Scheurleer, 281.

50 University of Oxford Archive, *Incorporation, NEP/ Supra Q, 10 July 1637, f.162v.*

Sir Thomas Browne, Shibden Dale and the Writing of *Religio Medici*

...I cannot forebear adding the learned Dr. Brown ...because in his Juvinal Years, he fixed himself in this Populous, and rich Trading Place, wherein to shew his Skill, and gain Respect in the World: And that during his Residence amongst us, and in his vacant Hours he writ his admired Peice, called by him Religio Medici. Dr. Samuel Midgely of Halifax, 1708[1]

The first literary work of Browne (Figure 5.1) was Religio Medici (RM) (Figure 5.2), an erudite reverie, composed after a classical education at Winchester College and Oxford University, followed by three years of medical studies at Montpellier, Padua, and Leiden.[2] Its publication in 1642 and 1643 (Figure 5.3) was an

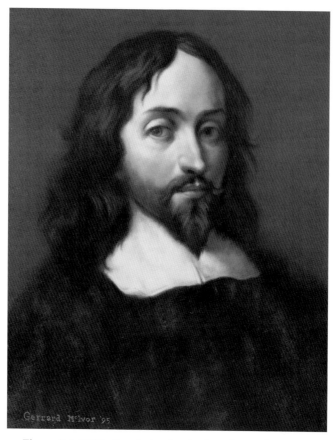

Figure 5.1 1995 oil painting by the late Gerrard McIvor, based on the engraving of Browne by David Loggan.

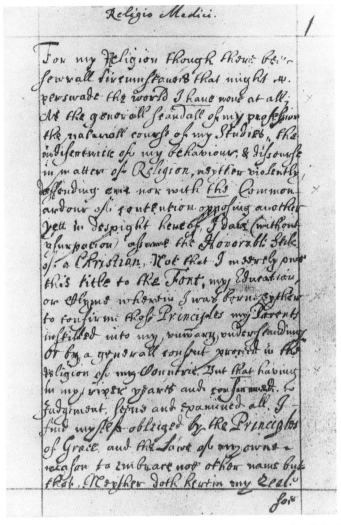

Figure 5.2 The first page of a 17th century manuscript copy of Religio Medici, one of two copies in the Norwich Library, and reproduced by their permission. Thought to be in the hand of Dr Reid, who died in 1641.

immediate success and the work has remained in print through scores of editions and translations. Many biographers and editors of Browne have pondered the place of writing.[3] This present account reviews the evidence that it was written in Shibden Dale, near Halifax, Yorkshire.

After receiving his doctorate of medicine in Leiden in December 1633, Browne returned to England to begin his medical career, but there was a legal difficulty: without an English MD, he could not practice as a physician. His Leiden degree could be 'incorporated' by Oxford (or Cambridge) University, and this took place in Oxford on July 10th 1637, the minimum period of fourteen years having intervened since his matriculation in Oxford in 1623. He then proceeded to

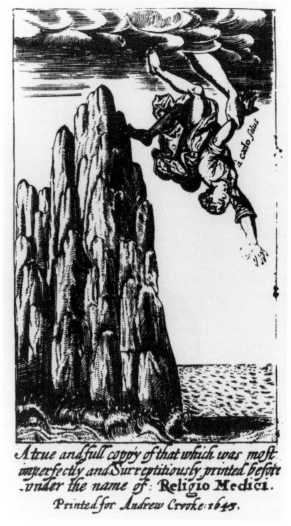

A true and full coppy of that which was most
imperfectly and Surreptitiously printed before
under the name of: Religio Medici.
Printed for Andrew Crooke: 1643.

Figure 5.3 Frontispiece of the 1643 (first authorized) edition of *Religio Medici*. Reproduced by permission from a copy in the Bodleian Library, Rawlinson 675.

Norwich for the remainder of a long career of medical practice. He spent the three years of 1634-1636 in gaining medical experience, choosing obscurity in the country. The Royal College of Physicians controlled practice in London and 'seven miles thereabouts', and, in Oxford, he would have been excluded from any substantial practice before 1637.

The date of composition may be calculated from the text: the manuscript was in existence in 1635, in which year, on October 19th, Browne was thirty. In part 1, section 41, he writes

'...*as yet I have not seen one revolution of Saturn, nor hath my pulse beat thirty years...*'.[4]

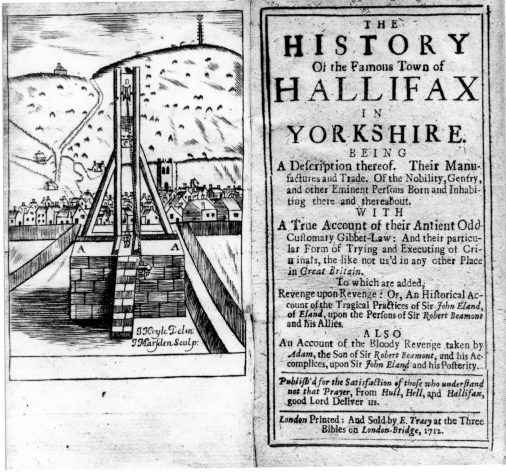

Figure 5.4 Frontispiece of the 1712 edition of History of Halifax. Reproduced by permission from a copy in the Bodleian Library, Douce B100.

Part 2 was written a little later for in section 11 he writes

'... *for my life, it is a miracle of thirty years, which to relate, were not a history, but a piece of poetry and would sound to common ears like a fable...*'.[5]

In the "Preface to the Reader" of the first authorized edition of 1643, he states that the work was composed seven years before.[6] We may conclude that the writing encompassed October 1635. Browne was moved by being thirty. In part 1, section 39 he writes

'... *some divines count Adam thirty years old at his creation, because they suppose him created in the perfect age and stature of man...*'.[7]

And later he writes:

'...*Let them not therfore complain of immaturity that die about thirty...*'.[8]

Where Religio Medici was written is less certain. London and Oxford are improbable, as Browne wrote in the "Preface to the Reader", that:

'... it was penned in such a place, and with such disadvantage, that (I protest) from the first setting of pen, to paper, I had not the assistance of any good book wherby to promote my invention or relieve my memory...'.[9]

Central to the evidence for Shibden Dale is Dr Samuel Midgley (c.1630-95), whose assertion begins this account. Midgley, of a prominent local family, was born some four or five years before Browne's residence in Yorkshire, and of him the Rev. Oliver Heywood, of Northowram, near Shibden Dale, minister at Colney Chapel in Halifax wrote in his Register:

'Samuel Midgly ...waited on us, hath been prisoner 3 times in Halifax jail for debt, dyed there, bur. July 18 '95, aged 66'.[10]

Midgely practised medicine but was frequently in debt, and, in Halifax jail, wrote *Hallifax and its Gibbet-Law Placed in a True Light*, which manuscript came to William Bentley, clerk of the Parish Church, who, 13 years after Midgely's death, published the book and appeared as the author. The 1712 edition in the Bodleian Library bears the inscription

'...Dr Samuel Midgely is said to have been the real author & to have written it when confined in Hallifax Gaol for Debt...'.

I see no reason to disbelieve Midgely's statement about Browne and the writing of RM: he was recollecting events in Halifax, when he was a child. Midgley writes amusingly, and claimed Browne as a medical and literary colleague. His book describes the Draconian treatment of miscreants in Halifax which prompted their prayer "From Hell, Hull, and Halifax, Good Lord deliver us". Stealing goods valued at more than thirteen pence and one halfpenny incurred the death penalty. I reproduce the title page and frontipiece of the 1712 edition of Midgley's book on the Gibbet-Law (Figure 5.4). The frontispiece is a chilling depiction of the method of execution in Halifax, which anticipated the introduction of Dr Guillotin's decapitating instrument in 1791.

Further corroboration of where RM was written is in Antiquities of the Parish of Halifax, by the Rev. Thomas Wright, formerly curate of the Parish Church. In 1712 Wright wrote:

'Neither must I omit in this Place Sir Thomas Browne, Doctor of Physick, who, tho' born in London, Oct. 19, 1605, yet practis'd here as a Physician in his younger Years. About the year 1630, he lived in Shipden Hall, nigh Halifax, at which time he wrote that excellent Piece, intitled Religio Medici.'[11]

Wright believed Midgley but the place was Over or Upper Shibden and his date of 1630 is a mistake. Browne obtained his degree in Leiden in 1633, having

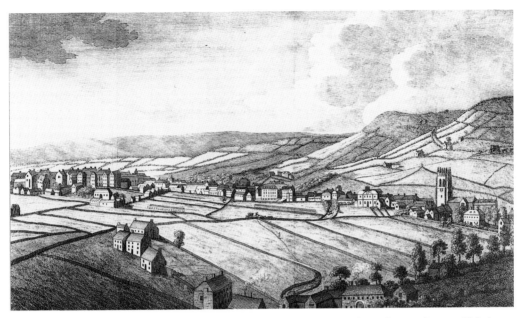

Figure 5.5 Engraving in Watson (1775) showing Halifax as seen from the South East. Shibden Dale extends to the right from the middle of the picture. Reproduced by permission from a copy in: the Bodleian Library, Gough Yorks 33 (2).

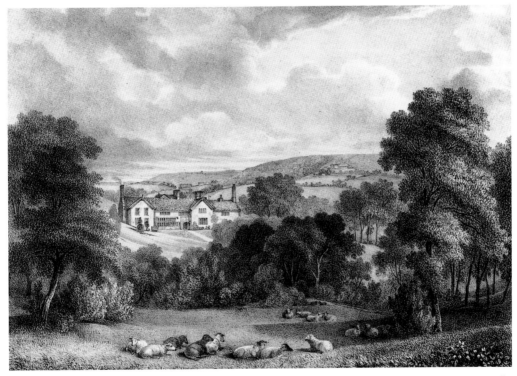

Figure 5.6 Lithograph by John Horner. dated 1835, of Shibden Hall, as viewed from Beacon Hill. Shibden Dale is behind and to the right of the Hall.

previously spent some three years on the continent of Europe. That he was in Halifax in 1630 is improbable.

The Reverend John Watson in his History and Antiquities of Halifax agreed with Midgley and Wright, and also described the families who owned and resided in Shibden Hall.[12] There were two halls of this name, Shibden Hall, occupied by Thomas Lister, but owned by a John Lister, who had purchased the house from Caleb Waterhouse, brother of Nathaniel, to whom I shall refer below (Figure 5.5). Higher up the valley was Upper or Over Shibden Hall which may have been Browne's residence. The building became a farmhouse, later was replaced by two cottages, and, early in the nineteenth century, was rebuilt in stone as the lodge of Upper Shibden Hall, built by the Stocks family.

When I visited in April 1999, Upper Shibden Hall and its Lodge were in ruins. The Reverend Bryan Dale, writing in 1896, visited the probable site in the company of Mr John Lister (1847-1933), then owner of Shibden Hall, and our main authority on where Browne resided in 1635 (Figure 5.6). They found a tenant in residence, a farm employee of Mr Michael Stocks of the Upper Shibden estate. Carved in stone over the fireplace of the kitchen, and surviving from the original old farmhouse, was the inscription J.S.F, 1626, a date about nine years before Browne's residence. The letters recall James Foxcroft and his wife Sarah. James Foxcroft was probably the brother of Anthony Foxcroft, who was the stepfather of Henry Power, also important in this quest.

The constables of Halifax are recorded in the Manuscripts of Mr J. Brearcliffe.[13] We note that '...*James Foxcroft of the Cross, formerly of [Upper] Shipden Hall...*' was constable in 1638-9. We may conclude that he built Upper Shipden Hall in 1626, and, before 1638, let it to someone because he moved to 'The Cross' as constable of Halifax. That someone was probably Browne.

This brings us to the Power family, and in particular to John Power, who was the son of William Power, Rector of Barwick.[14] For several generations the Power family sent their sons to Cambridge, after which the eldest became clergymen. John was the youngest of four sons, and was in trade – his sobriquet was *"the Spanish Merchant"*. In coming to Halifax, he joined his sister Ann, who had married John Favour, the Vicar of Halifax. John Power married Jane Jennings who bore him four sons and a daughter. Henry, the first born, (b.1623 or 1624), became a doctor, and later a frequent correspondent of Browne in Norwich.[15] When John died in 1638, Henry's mother married Anthony Foxcroft, who became Henry Power's stepfather. Anthony was the brother of James Foxcroft, the owner of Upper Shibden Hall. In a letter to Browne written from Halifax on June 13th, 1646, Henry Power gives an account of his studies at Cambridge, and adds the postscript

'. . . *our towne can furnish you with very small news, only the death of some of your acquaintance, viz., Mr Waterhouse and Mr. Sam Mitchell. . .*'[16]

Mr Waterhouse was Nathaniel Waterhouse, a prominent benefactor of Halifax.[17] At about the time of Browne's residence, he built the workhouse and obtained a *'Charter of Poor Law Incorporation'* in which Samuel Mitchell and John Power were two of the twelve governors. The death of Nathaniel Waterhouse, a "Salter and Oyl-Drawer", in August 1642, was a notable event in Halifax. The letter of Henry Power to Browne continues:

> *This enclos'd is from my Father-in-Law [Anthony Foxcroft] to your selfe: if your occasions will permitt the returne of a few lines to either of us by this bearer, wee shall be very glad to accept them.*[18]

Two years later Henry Power is again writing to Browne from Christ's College Cambridge:

> *Sr, My father Foxcroft & Mother, in their last to Cambridge forgott not to tender their best respects to you, wch I have requited in the like returne of yrs to them.*[19]

Only two letters from Browne to Power have survived, and that dated June 8, 1659 is significant.[20] By now Henry Power had obtained his medical degree, had married a daughter of Foxcroft by a previous marriage, and was living in New Hall, near Elland. The letter concludes:

> *Deare Sr, I wish my time would permitt my communication with you in any proportion to my desires, wherein I should never bee werie, wherby I might continue the delight I have formerely had by many serious discourses with my old friend, your good father [John Power], whose memorie is still fresh with mee, & becomes more delightful by this great enjoyment I have had from his true & worthy sonne.*

It is beyond doubt that Browne spent a significant period of time near Halifax and made an enduring acquaintanceship with several of the prominent families of the town. His main link to Halifax was the Power family, and possibly John Power was an old acquaintance. Correspondence to Browne from Halifax continued after the death of Henry Power in 1668.[21] John Brearcliffe, the Halifax antiquary, wrote 4 Aug: 1669 with a list of copies of Roman coins *'for his worthy friend Dr Browne'*.[22]

I make four conclusions on the foregoing evidence:

1. Religio Medici was written around the year 1635 when Browne began his thirtieth year.

2. At this time, Browne spent some time near Halifax, being acquainted with the Power family, Anthony Foxcroft, and local worthies such as Nathaniel Waterhouse, and Samuel Mitchell.

3. It is probable that he was a tenant of James Foxcroft in a building in Shibden Dale.

4. No alternate evidence having emerged, it is probable that part or all of Religio Medici was written in Shibden Dale and that this was where '...*I had not the assistance of any goode booke...*'

I give the evidence above in detail as one biographer, and some editors have disbelieved this location.[23] Of Browne's biographers, Simon Wilkin first put forward Shibden Hall, Halifax, quoting Bentley [Midgely], Wright, Watson, and Whitaker.[24] Bryan Dale agreed after painstaking enquiry.[25] Edmund Gosse, Jeremiah Finch, and Joan Bennett followed this general opinion. Samuel Johnson thought

'...*about the year 1634 he is supposed to have returned to London; and the next year to have written his celebrated treatise, called Religio Medici...*'

Johnson gives no authority for this statement, which, in any case, does not say that RM was written in London.[26] Professor Huntley, in his excellent literary study of Browne, questioned the location in Yorkshire, alternatively proposing Oxfordshire, quoting Wood.[27] I find Huntley's arguments unconvincing, and his reference to Wood inappropriate. The relevant passage states

'...*in the beginning of theyear 1623, [Browne] took the degrees in arts, as a member of the said coll. entred on the physic line, and practised that faculty for some time in these parts...*'[28]

Wood is silent on where Religio Medici was written. It seems unlikely that the book could have been written in or around Oxford, and that no account of its place of writing has survived. And again, anywhere near Oxford would ensure access to '*a goode booke*', the lack of which Browne 'protests'.

Why Browne spent a period in Halifax is unknown. There was no obvious family connection with Chester or London. Most of his schoolfellows at Winchester were from the south of England and often from near Winchester[29] Exceptions were John Hutton who entered in 1620, came from Richmond, and was the son of the Archbishop of York; and William Parker who entered in 1621 and was from Waddington, Yorkshire. Halifax had more numerous links with Oxford. Robert Clay of Merton College – one of the Clays of Clayhouse – was the Vicar of Halifax from 1623. He died in 1628 and was succeeded by Hugh Ramsden again of Merton. Hugh Ramsden's tenure was short as he died in 1629, to be succeeded by his brother Henry Ramsden, a graduate of Magdalen Hall and previously Fellow of Lincoln College, Oxford. Henry was Vicar during Browne's residence, and remained so until his death in 1637.

It is possible that during Browne's travels on the continent, and in his periods in Montpellier, Padua, and Leiden, he befriended someone from Yorkshire. There is a strong bond between Browne and the Power family: he knew John Power the Spanish Merchant from "...*many serious discourses.*" Browne read Spanish and Henry Power sent him 'old Spanish Bookes I have found of my Fathers'.[30] Henry was eleven or twelve in 1635, when Browne was in Halifax, and, exceptionally, chose medicine as a career, being the first physician in five generations of the Power family.[31] Henry proceeded to qualify in medicine at Cambridge, informally supervised by Browne, and becoming a lifelong friend and correspondent. We may yet discover with more certainty why Browne went to Halifax but, meanwhile the words of Samuel Midgley state that he did, and with benefit to literature.

ACKNOWLEDGEMENTS

I thank the staffs of the British, Bodleian and Halifax Libraries, and those of Shibden Hall, Halifax.

NOTES AND REFERENCES

[1] Midgley, S. *Hallifax and its Gibbet-Law Placed in a true Light*, printed by J. How for William Bentley, Hallifax, 1708. Further editions appeared in 1712, 1761, and 1789, and in 1886 a reprint of the 1708 edition was made by J. H. Turner of Bradford. My quotation (pp. 88-9) and illustration are from the 1712 edition, as 1708, but with a different title and frontispiece.

[2] References are from Browne, T. *The Works of Sir Thomas Browne* (henceforth *Works*), Vols. 1-6. Keynes, G, ed. London: Faber and Gwyer, becoming Faber and Faber, 1928-1931. RM is in vol. 1, 198.

[3] The place of writing is mentioned in: Johnson, S. 'Life', included in *Christian Morals* by Sir Thomas Browne of Norwich, MD. London: 1756; Wilkin, S. *The Works of Sir Thomas Browne*. London: Henry Bohn, 1835-6; Gosse, E. *Sir Thomas Browne*, London: Macmillan & Co, 1905; Finch, J.S. Sir Thomas Browne: *A Doctor's Life of Science and Faith* New York: Henry Schuman, Inc, 1950; Bennett, J. *Sir Thomas Browne: A Man of Achievement in Literature*, Cambridge: Cambridge University Press, 1962; Huntley, F.L. *Sir Thomas Browne: A Biographical and Critical Study*. Ann Arbor, USA: University of Michigan Press, 1968.

[4] *Works*, 1, 51.

[5] *Works*, 1, 91.

[6] There is a facsimile of the Bodleian Library copy of the 1643 (first authorized) edition of RM, (Menton, UK, Scolar Press, 1970).

[7] *Works*, 1, 49.

[8] *Works*, 1, p.53.

[9] RM. Preface'To the Reader'. In *Works*, 1, 4.

[10] Heywood, O. and Dickenson, T. *The Nonconformist Register* 1644-1750, ed. by J.H. Turner, Brighouse, J.S. Jowett, 1881, 80.

[11] Wright, T. *The Antiquities of the Town of Halifax in Yorkshire, etc.* Leeds: James Lister, 1738, 152. Reprint edited by J.H. Turner, Bingley: T.Harrison, 1884.

[12] Watson, J. *The History and Antiquities of the Parish of Halifax in Yorkshire*, London: T. Lowndes, 1775. Facsimile Didsbury, E.J. Morten, 1973.

[13] Brearcliffe's manuscripts are in Watson, J. *The History and Antiquities of the Parish of*

Halifax: enlarged, 2nd ed. London and Halifax, 1869-80. See also Watson, J. *Biographia Halfaxiensis or Halifax Families and Worthies*, Bingley: J.H. Turner, 1883.

[14] Clay, J.W. 'Dr Henry Power of New Hall, F.R.S.', *Papers and Reports of the Halifax Antiquary Society*, (1917), 1-31.

[15] British Library (henceforth BL) *MS. Sloane 1911-3*. The letters are reproduced in Halliwell, J.O.: '*A Collection of Letters of Science in England*'. London: Historical Society of Science, 1841, 913, and in Keynes, *Works*, VI, pp. 275-295.

[16] BL. *Sloane 1911-13, f.76*. In *Works*, 6, 280.

[17] Biographies of the Power, Foxcroft, Waterhouse, and Lister families are given in Watson, J. and Turner, J.H. *Biographia Halifaxiensis* Bingley: T. Harrison, 1883.

[18] *BL. Sloane 1911-13, f.76*. In *Works*, 6, 283-4.

[19] *BL. Sloane 1911-13, f.80*. In *Works*, 6, 283-4.

[20] *BL. Sloane 3515, f.60*. In *Works*, 6, 292-5.

[21] Henry Power died on Dec 23 in Wakefield, where he was buried. His will, dated Dec 19, 1668, was proved at York.

[22] Bodleian Library, Oxford. *MS Rawlinson D391, ff. 77-78*.

[23] Huntley, pp.90-7. Editors quoting Huntley are Keynes, G. *The Works of Sir Thomas Browne*, 2nd. ed. vols 1-4, London, Faber and Faber, 1964, 1, p.3, n.1; and Patrides, C.A. *Sir Thomas Browne: The Major Works*. London: Penguin Books, 1977, 60, n.5.

[24] Wilkin. *Supplementary Memoir*, 1, lviii-lix.

[25] Dale, B. 'Shibden Dale and Sir Thomas Browne's Religio Medici', *The Bradford Antiquary*, n.s. 1 (1896), 45-57.

[26] Johnson, p.v. The life is also in Wilkin, 1, p.xx.

[27] Huntley, 90-7.

[28] Wood, A. *Athenae Oxoniensis*. Vols 1-4, Bliss, P, ed. London: many publishers, 1813, 4, 56.

[29] Browne's schoolfellows at Winchester are given in Kirby, T.F. *Annals of Winchester College*, London: Henry Froude, and Winchester, P. and G. Wells, 1892.

[30] BL. *MS. Sloane 3515, f.59. Works*, 6, p.289.

[31] Thoresby, R. *Ducatus Leodiensis*. London: Maurice Atkins, 1715, 260.

Sir Thomas Browne's Knighthood

In September 1671, Browne was knighted in Norwich, deservedly but unexpectedly, as he was then 65 years of age, with no conspicuous activities to excite his sovereign. His earlier fame as the author of *Religio Medici* had receded, and though *Pseudodoxia Epidemica* was in its sixth English edition – to be the last in the author's lifetime –, it was, despite many revisions, outdated. To a select circle, *Hydrotaphia* and *The Garden of Cyrus*, published in 1658, gave pleasure, but would scarcely have been read by Charles II. In medical and scientific circles, Browne was known as a Fellow of the Royal College of Physicians and a frequent correspondent of the Royal Society to which, however, he did not belong. Browne's knighthood came from the chance of meeting his sovereign during the progress of King Charles through Norfolk. Descriptions of the scene by modern biographers of Browne have wrongly suggested that Browne was a substitute candidate for this honour.[1] The phrase 'gained by default' has been used.[2] Yet witness accounts and records provide an accurate portrayal the purpose of this communication.

Three contemporary accounts of the royal visit exist: a poem by Mathew Stevenson; a letter from Thomas Corie, the Town Clerk of Norwich; and a report in the *London Gazette*, dated Oct 1st, from the Court at Whitehall.[3] Mathew Stevenson (fl. 1654-1685), a poet of local renown, resided for the greater part of his life in Norfolk.[4] Thomas Corie was of a family prominent in Norwich for civic offices, and his part in this narrative is that of a correspondent to Joseph Williamson, founder and editor of the *London Gazette*.[5] The verse quotations below are from the poet whilst those in prose, without separate identification, derive from the letter of Thomas Corie. Records of the corporations of Yarmouth and Norwich refer to the event.[6] There are also relevant references in state papers.[7] The account in Echard is mainly derived from the *London Gazette*.[8] That of Blomefield is widely quoted, but has been misread, as was noted by Ketton-Cremer.[9]

Royal visits to Norwich and Norfolk were rare, and that of Queen Elizabeth, in the summer of 1578, was long remembered by the citizens of Norwich.[10] Throughout a whole week, a succession of masques, pageants, and banquets, punctuated with Latin orations, gave evidence of the rapturous enthusiasm of the Norwich burghers for their queen, who, on departing, exclaimed 'I have laid up in my breast such good will, as I shall never forget Norwich.[11]

The progress of Charles was similarly welcomed although the tastes and purpose of this sovereign differed. It was the first visit of Charles to Norfolk and its timing was important politically and strategically. He had recently visited

Portsmouth, the Isle of Wight, and Plymouth. For reasons more venial than religious, Charles was considering conversion to Roman Catholicism, and he was also in the company of a new mistress. Charles was contemplating war with the Dutch and, in May 1670, the secret Treaty of Dover had been signed by Charles' Catholic ministers.[12] The signatories of the sham Treaty of Dover later in 1670 included others, notably his Protestant minister, Ashley. Both treaties united Great Britain and France in a war against the United Provinces, which was declared by the King in Council on March 17th, 1672.[13] What Charles gained from the secret treaty was money from Louis XIV – immediate and deferred – in return for an alliance with France and his conversion to Catholicism, the latter condition being prominent in the secret treaty, but absent from the sham treaty. France wanted the alliance to combat the Dutch at sea and the money was to be spent on the English navy[14] Charles preferred this secret subsidy from Louis to an appeal to Parliament for funds.[15]

These national considerations clarify the timing of the progress into Norfolk and the visit by Charles and his brother James, the Lord High Admiral, to Yarmouth, a visit planned as early as April 20 1670.[16] The visit, arranged for April, 1671, had been abruptly postponed because of the death of the Duchess of York on March 31 of that year.[17] State records at this time abound with expenditure on the navy, and Yarmouth was an important port in naval actions against the Dutch.[18] Moreover Yarmouth, in common with many seaports, had been damaged by a great storm on September 11th and 12th, described as 'the most violent storms & rains within the memory of man'.[19] On Sept 18th many ships were reported lost in Yarmouth: 'We are already informed of fourteen sail of this town, and fear many more, beside the loss in the fishery'.[20]

The King came to Norfolk from Newmarket, where he frequently stayed to indulge in racing, hunting, and hawking. On Tuesday the 26th of September the royal party of King and Queen with many attendants left Newmarket for Euston House in Suffolk, the splendid new house of Lord and Lady Arlington. The king's stay was enhanced by the presence of his new mistress, Louise de Keroualle, a lovely diminutive Breton lady, who had waited on his sister Minette at Dover. This novelty was not free from international intrigue. To further the alliance and the conversion of Charles to catholism, the lady was recommended to the king by Colbert, the French Ambassador.

On the second day, the 27th, the King, his brother James, and the Dukes of Monmouth and Buckingham set out for Yarmouth, whilst the Queen remained for a further night at Euston House with her hosts and the most recent royal mistress. King and train broke their fast at the White Hart at Scole and by 5 o'clock arrived in Yarmouth, to a tumultous welcome of canonade, cheers, and loyal addresses. The Corporation presented the king with four gold herrings with ruby eyes and a gold chain[21] The king knighted the Recorder and the two Bailiffs and possibly one other, since Stevenson wrote. 'They say his Majesty there knighted Four, I only wonder he did knight no more.' The town was inspected and then the port and ships. Twelve hundred guns were fired and Charles named a new ship James after his brother. At the banquet in the evening, Yarmouth did in the poet's words 'entertain, season providing dishes, The King of England, with the King of Fishes'. Typically, Charles ate with relish from the dish of herrings served to him, 'All pleased the King, and the King did all please'.

Norwich awaited the royals in the afternoon of Thursday the 28th September at one o'clock, the reception party being the Mayor, Sheriff, and Aldermen, the Bishop, Dean, and Chapter with local clergy, and the party of Lord Henry Howard, 'Then highborn Howard waits the King's approaches, with's prancing horses, and his Prince's Coaches'. They were in some difficulty, as the King was to arrive first over Trowse bridge, whilst the Queen, coming further, from Euston, would cross Cringleford bridge, and possibly could be met later. As such arrangements frequently turn out, the King was late, arriving at 4 o'clock and the recorder, Francis Corie, afforced by the sons of Lord Henry, had to divert to Cringleford bridge in pursuit of the Queen and company, who had attained 'halfe a myle' into the city. To compound their troubles it had rained for several hours. Nevertheless the King, at Trowse bridge, was welcomed by a speech from the mayor, and a present worth 200 guineas, whilst the Queen was greeted by the second company. The couple were united at the Palace of the Duke of Norfolk, to which they were separately conducted through welcoming crowds lined by 200 liverymen and 700 soldiers of the City Regiment.

Thomas Fuller described the Palace as 'Amongst private houses, the Duke of Norfolk's Palace is the greatest I ever saw in a City out of London' and praised the 'covered bowling alley, the first I believe of that kind in England'.[22] Evelyn was less impressed by the architecture which he described as:

> an old wretched building, and that part of it newly built of brick, is ill understood; so as I was of opinion it had been much better to have demolished all, and set it up in a better place.

But for size, splendour, and luxury the house was unrivalled in East Anglia and, for this munificence in entertainment, Norwich was indebted to the family of the Duke of Norfolk.[24] At the palace, Lord Henry Howard deputised for his brother, the Duke of Norfolk who, not in possession of his senses, lived a retired life in Padua. Henry Howard had less than a months notice of his royal guests and had '...to post hither out of Yorkshire, to prepare here for all this vast reception...'. The resources of the palace were fully engaged. In addition to the train of the King, the Queen had a retinue of 55 persons, and all were accommodated in the great Palace, where,

> all the house through out was nobilie & richlie furnished with bedds, hangings, & ye apurtenances for lodging. The old Tennis-court turn'd into a kitchen, and

ye Duke's bowlinge alley (which as ye know is one hundred & thirty foote wyde & one hundred & nyntye foote long) made into sevrall roomes for eateinge.

That night the scale of the banquet exceeded any former occasion in the Palace, 'none who did not see it can well express the splendour of it'[25]

Charles was busy the following day, beginning with touching for the King's evil. This condition was bovine tuberculosls manifest as swelling of the lymph glands of the neck, and arising from by the ingestion of tubercle bacilli from water or milk. It was widely believed that this condition was amenable to the touch of the king, and physicians provided certificates admitting their patients to the presence of the king. Browne frequently provided these certificates, the usual circumstance being a visit of the king to Newmarket.[26]

The King then was driven to the Cathedral where he was 'sung into the church with an anthem'. After his devotions, he went to the neighbouring Bishop's Palace 'to refresh himselfe with a glass of choyce wyne & sweetmeates'. After a brief return to the Duke's Palace, he was conducted to the Guild Hall, where 'he had from the leads a prospect of ye City, & saw our whole Regt in armes with thier redd-coates' and showed himself to the joyous citizens who 'soe filled ye whole Market-place, as his Majesties coach had scarse roome to passe thence to the New Hall'. The New Hall had been the nave of the Church of the Dominican Black Friars, and, after the Reformation, had become an assembly hall, used for civlc function.[27] At the New Hall the King joined the Queen and 'received a noble treate from ye City', which included a great reception. The response of the King was to confer a knighthood. In the words of Blomefield:

> When his Majesty was at the New-Hall, he was earnest to have knighted the Mayor [Thomas Thacker], who as earnestly begged to be excused; but at the same time conferred the honour on that deserving physlclan Dr.Thomas Browne...[28]

The report from the Court in the London Gazette reads: 'And at Norwich was pleased to confer the same honor (knighthood] on the famous Dr. Browne'.[29] Echard restates this as 'And before the King parted from the city, he conferr'd the honour of knighthood upon the famous physician, Dr Thomas Browne'.[30]

The morning had so far been busy and it was now eleven o'clock.[31] Their majesties and his royal highness and other members of the court entered their coaches to drive to the house of Sir John Hobart at Blickling some miles to the North. There, dinner was taken, the visit exemplifying Charles' diplomacy, for Sir John Hobart was a notable Puritan, and had married a daughter of John Hampden. Sir John had been a Cromwellian, supporting the Lord Protector in the County, in the House of Commons, and in the short-lived Upper House. The guests at Blickling were 'most noblie and plentifully treated' and Charles responded with a knighthood to Sir John's son. All was polite and gracious but it was unlikely that

King and Court would overnight in this puritan household. The Queen and her company returned to the ducal palace at Norwich, whilst the King and his entourage drove for the night to Oxnead, the great house of his supporter, Sir Robert Paston. So ended the Progress and the visit to Norwich which in the closing words of Stevenson, 'Norwich strained all, that Norwich cou'd extend, Nor cou'd she more, should Jove himself descend'.

The account above quotes contemporary evidence and should be compared with that of modern biographers. Johnson gave no details of the occasion but commended the King who 'with many frailties and vices, had yet skill to discover excellence, and virtue to reward it, with such honorary distinctions as cost him nothing'[32] This penetrating opinion exactly grasps the character of Charles, whose many foolish actions were mingled with others showing discernment. This opinion was that expressed by Joan Bennett in her study of Browne's literary merit.[33] Gosse wrote

> He was proceeding to confer this honour to Thomas Thacker, the mayor, when that worthy modestly and humbly begged that it might be given to the most eminent inhabitant of the city, indicating the author of Religio Medici.

Gosse also believed that the King visited Browne's house and observed him dissecting a dolphin, this error arising from a letter of Browne to his son. Browne merely wrote 'You may remember the dolphin opened when the King was heere'.[35] It is the imagined incident of the mayor's decline of the honour and proposing that it be bestowed on Browne, first described by Gosse, which is so frequently repeated, by Leroy, Finch and Huntley. Finch described a pretty scene:

> The much-feted monarch had arisen to propose... the knighting of the Mayor, Mr. Henry Herne. But at this point Herne 'earnestly begged to be excused' ...A whispered consultation produced a solution. The name of Dr. Thomas Browne was called, and all eyes turned toward the physician, whose sensitive face, framed by rich brown hair, seemed more than usually meditative as he gravely approached the King, kneeled, and arose a knight.[36]

Huntley writes

> Toward the end of the toasts, the king, as was his custom, proposed to knight the mayor of the city, one Mr Henry Herne. But the mayor 'earnestly begged to be excused' and suggested in his stead Norwich's most famous citizen, Dr Thomas Browne.'[37]

In the witness reports, that I have examined, there is no evidence of this scene, and the mayor, in 1671, was Mr Thomas Thacker, not Hearne, the mayor in 1673.[38]

My account exemplifies how capriciously knighthoods were bestowed by the Stuart Kings. Elizabeth had been frugal with honours and there were some 500 knights on the accession of James 1.[39] James immediately began to create knights on a scale hitherto unknown. The sale of knighthoods by the King and his courtiers was disreputable, and the rank of knighthood lost esteem. A popular jest described two walkers observing another 'the one demanded what he should be, the other answered he seemed to be a gentleman; no I warrant you, says the other, I think he is but a knight'.[40] Charles II was similarly immoderate in the number of knights he created, and on this Progress, he created four in Yarmouth and several more in Norwich. The following day, at Blickling, he knighted Henry Hobart, who, at the age of thirteen, seems a young recipient and, as the eldest son of Sir John Hobart, would, in any case, have expected to inherit his father's baronetcy. Amongst this widespread knightage in the Stuart period, the number of doctors so honoured is small. William Harvey, despite loyal service as physician to three kings, did not receive a knighthood, nor did Francis Glisson, Thomas Sydenham, or Thomas Willis. Besides Sir Thomas Browne, Sir George Ent and Sir William Petty were notable medical knights, but Petty was more active as a scientist and political economist than as a physician. Opinions on the life of Charles II are divided. Mine is that, on balance, and there is a lot to forgive, he was an able king. But we must all commend his act in the New Hall, at Norwich, on the morning of Friday, September 29th, 1671. The poet commended his city and his king:

> And now with Norwich, for whose sake I writ,
> Let me conclude; Norwich did what was fit:
> Or, what with them was possible, at least;
> That City does enuff, that does its best.
> There the King knighted the so famous Brown, whose worth,
> & learning to the world are known.

Browne was a worthy recipient of a knighthood, which was widely commended, and, in subsequent centuries, remembers an outstanding individual with a common given and a common family name. Many have borne the name Thomas Browne, but Sir Thomas Browne brings only one person to mind.

NOTES AND REFERENCES

[1] Biographers who have described the scene are: Edmund Gosse, *Sir Thomas Browne.* London: 1905, 160-1; Olivier Leroy, *Le Chevalier Thomas Browne.* Paris: 1931, 76-7; Jeremiah S. Finch, *Sir Thomas Browne.* New York: Macmillan, 218-9; Frank L. Huntley, *Sir Thomas Browne.* (Ann Arbor, University of Michigan Press: 1962, 1968), 242-243.

[2] C.A. Patrides, ed., *Sir Thomas Browne, The Major Works.* London: Penguin Press 1977, 21.

[3] Mathew Stevenson, 'Upon His Majesties Progress into Norfolk, Sept 28 1671', In *Norfolk Drollery.* London: 1673, 23-30; 'Coppie of a Letter from T.C. [Thomas Corie] at Norwich to a Friend [Joseph Williamson] in London, Norwich, October ye 2d, 1671', British Library, *Add MSS 27,967, f 88*; *The London Gazette.* London (1671), No 613, Sept 24-Oct 2, 2.

[4] *Dictionary of National Biography*. London: 1909, 18, 1129-1130.

[5] Robert H. Hill, ed. 'The Correspondence of Thomas Corie, Town Clerk of Norwich, 1664-1687', *Norfolk Record Society Publ. (1956)*, Norwich, VII. The letter to Joseph Stevenson, then editor of the London Gazette is reproduced.

[6] Relevant entries in the Yarmouth and Norwich Corporation Books are reproduced in Dawson Turner, *Narrative of the visit of His Majesty King Charles the Second to Norwich*. Yarmouth: 1846.

[7] *Calendar of State Papers, Venice (CSPV)* and *Calendar of State Papers, Domestic (CSPD)*. London: 1939, 1895.

[8] Laurence Echard, *The History of England from the Restoration . . Queen Mary*. London: 1707-18 vol 3, book 1, chapter 3, 281.

[9] Francis Blomefield, *History of Norfolk, 10 vols*. London: 1805-10, 3, 413-4; R.W. Ketton Cremer, 'The Visit of King Charles the Second to Norfolk', In *Norfolk Portraits*. London: 1944, 14n.

[10] John Nichols, *The Progresses and Public Processions of Queen Elizabeth* 3 vols. London: 1823, 2, 133-178.

[11] Nichols, 166.

[12] Echard, 253 4.

[13] Echard, 294-5.

[14] *CSPV*, London, 1939, 37, 113. Oct.3rd, 1671. The Doge was informed by Girolami Alberti, Venetian Secretary in England, that the King is 'to fit out a fleet by means of a monthly assignment of 60,000 1'. Alberti suspected that Charles had received 'a considerable sum of money', enabling him to dissolve parliament.

[15] Announced from the Court on Sept. 23rd, 1671 in the *London Gazette*.

[16] Yarmouth Corporation Book, April 20, 1670. Reproduced in Dawson Turner, above.

[17] *CSPD*, 1671, 70, 170. HRH died on April 3rd.

[18] *CSPD*, many references in 1671.

[19] *CSPD*, 1671, 480.

[20] *CSPD*, 1671, 488.

[21] Yarmouth Corporation Book, *Sept. 18th, 1671*, and *CSPD*, 1671, 70, 488.

[22] Thomas Fuller, *The History of the Worthies of England*, ed., John Nichols 2 vols. London: 1811, 2, 154.

[23] John Evelyn, *Diary* 3 vols. London: 1906, 2, 334.

[24] Described in Ernest A. Kent, 'The Houses of the Dukes of Norfolk in Norwich', *Norfolk Archaeology*, Norwich, 24 (1931), 73-87.

[25] B.L., Add MSS 27,967, f88. Reproduced in Hill. Appended to Thomas Corie's letter is a list of the persons accompanying the King and Queen.

[26] Letter from Sir Thomas Browne to his son Edward, dated Oct. 2,[1679], British Library, *MS 1847, f.217*.

[27] Antony Batty Shaw, *Sir Thomas Browne of Norwich*. Norwich: 1982, fig. 29.

[28] This text is from Blomefield, 3, 413-414, and does not state that the mayor suggested Browne as a substitute.

[29] *The London Gazette*, 1671, 613, Sept.24-Oct.2, 2.

[30] Echard, 281.

[31] It was a morning, not an evening, reception at the New Hall.

[32] Samuel Johnson, 'The Life of Sir Thomas Browne', In, *Christian Morals*. (London: 1756), xxxvi.

[33] Bennett J, *Sir Thomas Browne, A man of achievement in literature*. Cambridge: Cambridge University Press 1962, 22.

[34] Gosse, 160-1.

[35] B.L., *MS Sloane 1847, f.98.*

[36] Finch, 218.

[37] Huntley, 242-3.

[38] Blomefield, 3, 420 ; Basil Cozens-Hardy & Ernest A. Kent, *The Mayors of Norwich*, 1403-1835. Norwich: 1938, 94 & 95.

[39] F.J. Fisher, ed., *The State of England, Anno Dom. 1600, by Thomas Wilson*. London: Camden Soc., 3rd ser., Lil, 1936 1-47.

[40] Barry Coward, *The Stuart Age*. London: 1980, 123.

Henry Power (1626-1668) of New Hall, Elland and Experiments on Barometric Pressure

The 6 of May, 1653. I took two Tubes, one of 45. inches, the other 35½ in length, and of different Diameters; and filling them both at the Bottom of *Hallifax-Hill*, the Quicksilver in both came down to its wonted pitch of 29.inches, thence going immediately to the top of the said Hill, and repeating the Experiment again, we found it there to fall more than half an inch lower[1]

On 6 May 1653, Henry Power conducted an historic experiment on Halifax Hill, demonstrating that the level of a mercury column operated as an altimeter. Ten years later, with Richard Townley, he made further barometric measurements and calculations, which, made before publication by Robert Boyle, demonstrated 'Boyle's Law'.[2] Henry Power was distinguished both in medicine and science and was an early member of the Royal Society.[3] His undeserved obscurity is explained by his early death at the age of forty two years, and the fact that, of his many writings, only *Experimental Philosophy* was published. This book contained, in addition to the barometric experiments to be narrated here, the first English work on microscopy, published before that of Robert Hooke. Power began his experiments in Cambridge, but his most important work was conducted at New Hall, Elland near Halifax, and in collaboration with Richard Townley at Townley in Lancashire. This present account focuses on his barometric experiments which began in Cambridge and continued in Elland near Halifax.

The Power family

The Power family bore arms in the reign of Henry VIII, when Francis Power married a daughter of the Bossevile family of New Hall.[4] This alliance began the association of the Power family with New Hall, built by the Saville family in the fifteenth century.[5] Of their three sons, we are concerned with William, whose son, another William, was Rector of Barwick in Elmet, West Riding from 1569-1594. His son – yet another William – became Lady Margaret Preacher at Cambridge. It was the second son, John Power, a wealthy manufacturer and trader in Halifax, known as the 'Spanish Merchant', who married Jane Jennings and was the father of our Henry Power. John had travelled widely and befriended Sir Thomas Browne who studied medicine at Montpellier, which contact may explain why Browne came to Halifax, where he wrote *Religio Medici*, a treatise possibly dedicated to John Power.[6] Henry whilst a child met Browne, who directed him to a career in medicine and science. He was the first doctor in the Power family, many generations of which had been clergymen. Henry Power was born in Annesley,

Notts in 1623 or 1626, probably the latter.[7] After schooling in Halifax, during which time his father died in 1638, he entered Christ's College, Cambridge as a pensioner on 15 December 1641.[8] Christ's was the college where his grandfather, William Power, had studied and where his uncle, another William Power, was the Senior Fellow and a prominent high churchman, leading a group in the college called the 'Powritians', detested by the Puritans in Cambridge.[9]

Experiments on Barometric Pressure in Renaissance Europe

The invention of the mercury barometer has been researched by Cornelis de Waard, to whose work, and to that of Knowles Middleton, I am indebted.[10] The discovery of Boyle's law by researchers in England has been explored by Webster.[11] In the early seventeenth century the existence of a vacuum, postulated by Democritus but denied by Aristotle, was gaining acceptance, despite objections of the Catholic Church. Also debated was that air had weight, could exert pressure and could be compressed. By 1612 Galileo had come to believe in the possibility of a vacuum, but did not believe that air had weight and could exert pressure, for in 1615 he was writing (translated): 'the air in itself and above the water weighs nothing'.[12] Isaac Beeckman (1588-1637), descended from a Cornelius Beeckman in Cologne, was sceptical.[13] In Caen, Beeckman was studying air pressure in the action of a suction pump, and defended his views in his MD thesis at the University of Caen.[14] In his journal he wrote (translated from Latin) 'air, after the manner of water, presses on things and compresses them according the depth of the superincumbent air'.[15] On 1 October 1629, Beeckman communicated his findings to Father Marin Mersenne in Paris.[16] Mersenne excelled as a collector and disseminator of research findings. Other researchers in France, *e.g.* Jean Rey, believed that air had weight and could exert pressure.[17]

We now come to decisive research in Italy. In Genoa, Giovanni Batista Baliani (1582-1666) observed that a siphon would not carry water over a hill which was twenty one metres above the supplying reservoir. If the siphon was filled with water and the ends opened, the water level dropped to about ten metres below the level of the upper reservoir. Baliani wrote to Galileo on 27 July 1630 in deferential manner – he was addressing the greatest living scientist – and Galileo replied promptly on 6 August.[18] His explanation was curious : a vacuum could have a force (*forza o resistenza del vacuo*). Galileo believed that a column of water required tensile strength, as did a pillar of stone or a post of wood.[19] As the length of the water column increased, its weight exceeded its strength and the column parted. Baliani was not satisfied with Galileo's reply and wrote again at length on 4 October.[20] The height of water possible in a syphon was also the limit of height in a suction pump, described in France by Beeckman, but this work was probably unknown in Italy.

The next advance, of great importance, took place in Rome among a group of scientists, which included Raffael Magiotti (1597-1658), Evangelista Torricelli

(1608-1647) and Gasparo Berti. They were stimulated by Galileo's *Discorsi* which, published in 1638, included the account from Baliani and Galileo's reply. Berti, from Mantua, a mathematician and astronomer, was a modest young man, who left few writings.[21] However there are four accounts, of which the most accurate is that of Emmanuel Maignan (1601-1676), who taught at the Convent on Monte Pincio in Rome and, some years later, returning to his native Toulose, wrote a long treatise on natural philosophy, which includes an account of the experiment.[22]

Gaspar Berti erected a leaden tube on the wall of his house, the upper end opposite a window, the lower end within a cask filled with water on the ground. The tube was filled with water and opening the brass tap below allowed water to attain a level seen in a flask fitted to the open upper brass tap. The water stood in the flask about 18 cubits. Berti and his colleagues had produced a vacuum, a concept denied by the Catholic Church, which explains why no contemporary accounts of the experiment exist. The date of the experiments may be estimated by a letter dated 12 March 1648, from Magiotti in Rome to Mersenne in Paris.[23] This includes the phrase (translated from Italian): 'Berti believed that he could convince Galileo with this experiment'.[24] So Galileo was still alive and the experiment preceded Galileo's death on 8 January 1642. The date was probably 1641.

Another observer of Berti's experiment in Rome was Torricelli, who in Florence planned a similar experiment using a glass tube filled with mercury.[25] The use of mercury had been suggested by Galileo and also by Viviani, a colleague of Torricelli in Florence. A copy of Galileo's 1638 *Discorsi* in Florence has marginal notes in the hand of Viviani where Galileo writes (translated):

And it is my belief that the same result will follow in other liquids, such as quicksilver... in which the rupture will take place to a lesser or greater height than 18 cubits, according to the ...specific gravity of these liquids[26]

Galileo still thought that the water column parted because its length exceeded its strength. The first mercury experiments are ascribed to Torricelli, but Viviani had the tubes constructed, obtained the mercury and performed the experiments, probably in 1644.[27] However, Torricelli is rightly considered the inventor of the barometer. His correspondence with Michelangelo Ricci in Rome shows an advanced knowledge of his experiment and the future uses of the mercury column, which he calls an instrument.[28]

Experiments on barometric pressure in France

The mercury experiments of Torricelli became generally known in France, probably from the traveller Balthasar de Monconys (1611-1665).[29] Again Mersenne is important, as he visited Florence in 1645 to see the experiment. Pierre Petit (1589-1677) performed the first experiment in France, at Rouen in 1646.[30] The group in Paris included Giles Persone de Roberval (1602-1675) and Blaise Pascal (1623-1662). Pascal reasoned that the mercury column, being maintained by air pressure, would be lower at higher altitude, which hypothesis he tested on a church steeple in Paris. His results were inconclusive because of the modest difference in height, and he proceeded to an historic experiment on the *Puy de Dome*, a high mountain in Auverne, near Clermont.

The experiment was performed by Pascal's brother-in-law, Florin Perier, on 19 September 1648 and was entirely successful. Two identical glass tubes 4 feet long, each sealed at one end, were filled with mercury and inverted into a vessel containing mercury. The level of the mercury in both was observed to be 26 inches and 3.5 lines. One tube remained in Clermont, whilst the other was carried to the top of the Puy de Dome, filled with mercury and inverted as before, when the mercury level was observed to be 23 inches and 2 lines, a drop of 3 inches and 1.5 lines. Meanwhile, the level in the tube at Clermont had not changed. Pascal wrote an account of this experiment in 1648.[31] However, it was not generally known until 1651 when the anatomist Jean Pecquet published his *Experimenta nova anatomica*.[32] Reading this work prompted Power to confirm the experiments of Pascal in Halifax in 1653. His work preceded that in Oxford and London. The Scot, George Sinclair, working in Glasgow, published in 1669.[33]

Experiments on barometric pressure in England

Knowledge of the Torricellian Experiment, with variations, passed by travellers and correspondents from Mersenne's circle in Paris to England.[34] Samuel Hartlib (c. 1600-1670) was a frequent correspondent of Mersenne. Sir Charles Cavendish (1591-1654), exiled in Paris during the Civil War, describes the experiment in a letter to William Petty dated April 1648.

> they prepare a long tube …which is filled with quicksilver …and being stopped by ones finger the tube is inverted and plunged in a vessel halfe or more full of quicksilver. The quicksilver in ye tube will force ye quicksilver in ye vessel to rise …and so leaves a space in ye top of the tube vacuum as is supposed[35]

There are frequent reports of the 'mercury experiment', and many variations were performed in London, Cambridge and Oxford. Wherever a group of philosophers gathered, they were fascinated by the properties of the vacuum above the mercury level. It was at Cambridge that Power, as a medical student, became acquainted with these experiments with mercury.

Henry Power at Cambridge

Power matriculated at Christ's College on 8 June 1641 and began his studies towards his BA, the subjects being the seven liberal arts: Grammar, Logic, Rhetoric, Arithmetic, Geometry, Astronomy and Music. Cambridge was a small town of less than 8000 inhabitants, isolated, swamp ridden, with endemic malaria and smallpox, and outbreaks of plague.[36] The students of the fifteen colleges numbered about 2,500, most of whom were destined for the church. Power's studies must have been curtailed by the Civil Wars, though Cambridge was less

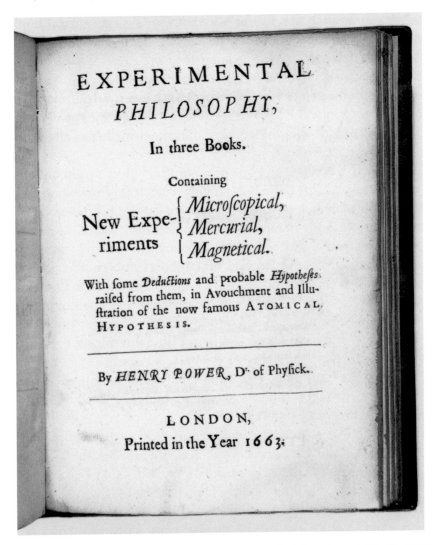

Figure 7.1 Title page of Book 2 of Power's *Experimental Philosophy*, published in 1663. From a copy in the possession of the author, as are figs. 3 & 4.

affected than Oxford. He gained his BA in 1645, in which year the first Civil War ended at the Battle of Naseby. The Puritans began a reform of Cambridge University and the Earl of Manchester came to enforce an ordinance of 22 January 1644. The Master of Christ's survived, but several fellows were ejected, amongst them William Power, the uncle of Henry. Both College and University were much altered when Power began his medical studies towards his MD.

The medical course required six years' residence, attendance at statutory lectures, viewing of two dissections, and disputations. At first sight, medical instruction at Cambridge seems negligible, being solely undertaken by the Regius Professor of Physic, who lectured four days a week on Hippocrates and Galen.[37]

Power was fortunate that the Regius was Francis Glisson, a notable physician, anatomist and physiologist. Glisson in his early years was a worthy teacher and later he was much in London and prominent in the Royal College of Physicians and the Royal Society.[38]   However, tuition was supplemented in the colleges by fellows qualified in medicine, who, ignoring the statutes, taught modern subjects in which they were interested. Christ's College, chosen by Power from family connections, was one of four colleges prominent in medicine, the others being Caius, St John's and Emmanuel.

In commencing his medical and scientific studies, Power sought advice from Dr Browne in Norwich.[39] This came in a famous letter from Browne in 1646 setting out a comprehensive course of study.[40] Scores of books in Browne's library were recommended for the study of medical practice, materia medica, anatomy, botany, zoology and chemistry. Browne seemed oblivious of the quantity of his recommended reading when he wrote: 'Although I mention but few books ...yet it is not my intention to confine you.' Power's correspondence with Browne was that of an apt pupil, determined to master both medicine and science. He valued his contact with Browne as much as his tutors in Cambridge, for on 15 September 1648 he is writing, 'Sr, I have a great desire to shift my residence a while & to live a moneth or two in Norwich by you'.[41]

Medical tuition at Cambridge was meagre but contacts with the Continent, in particular France, brought modern medicine and science to Cambridge. In philosophy, Platonism was prominent.

The Cambridge Platonists included Benjamin Whichcote (1609-1683), Henry More (1614-1687), Ralph Cudworth (1617-1688), and John Smith (1618-1682).[42] Henry Moore was a fellow of Christ's from 1639, and Ralph Cudworth, formerly Fellow of Emmanuel and Master of Clare Hall, became Master of Christ's in 1654. The philosophy of Descartes at first interested the Platonists, but later they saw that Cartesianism could not be reconciled with Platonism. Moore initially welcomed the views of Descartes, but later violently opposed them. To Power's medical studies, Cartesian science added observations in anatomy, physiology, botany and zoology, and also experiments. The mercury experiments were of particular interest and these Power began performing himself, in Cambridge and in Halifax, in the years before obtaining his MD in 1655. This was a fruitful period of research as, after 1655, he was occupied with his practice as a physician in Halifax.

Henry Power's writings

Power's early death curtailed the publication of much of his research, but a substantial body of manuscripts is preserved in the British Library. There are three manuscript versions of his barometric research at Cambridge and Halifax, two in the British Library and one in the Bodleian Library.[43] The Bodleian *MS* is a copy

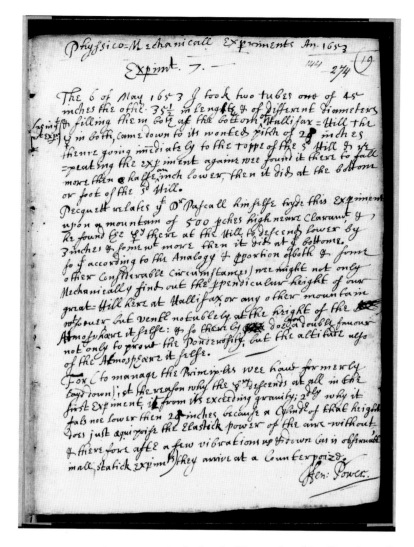

Figure 7.2 Signed manuscript in the hand of Power, describing Experiment 7.
Reproduced by permission of the Britsh Library, *Sloane Ms. 1393, folio 144, recto.*

of the original notes of the experiments made, according to a note on the *MS*, by 'John Sponge'. Mr John Spong (b. 1623) was a mathematician and instrument maker in London. The Sloane *MS 1333* is a bound notebook of a military engineer, to which is appended a shortened, incomplete version in Latin of Power's barometric experiments. *Sloane MS 1393* (Figure 7.2) is the version from which the 1663 *Experimental Philosophy* was printed. It is in Power's hand, with minor corrections and additions, and almost every page is signed. Comparison with the book shows that further changes were made, possibly in proof. For example, Torricellus is described in the *MS* as the 'French Engineer', but becomes the 'eminent Mathematician' in the book.

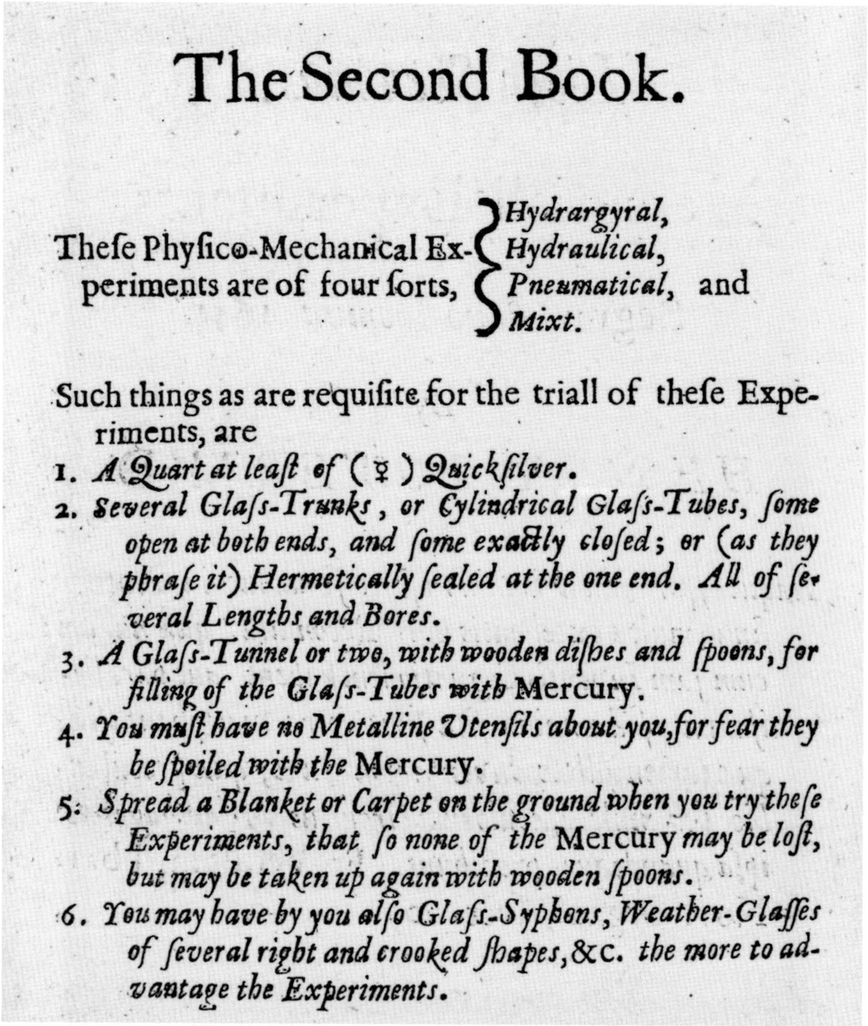

The Second Book.

Thefe Phyfico-Mechanical Ex- { *Hydrargyral,*
periments are of four forts, { *Hydraulical,*
{ *Pneumatical,* and
{ *Mixt.*

Such things as are requifite for the triall of thefe Experiments, are

1. *A Quart at leaft of* (☿) *Quickfilver.*
2. *Several Glafs-Trunks , or Cylindrical Glafs-Tubes, fome*
open at both ends, and fome exactly clofed; or (as they
phrafe it) Hermetically fealed at the one end. All of fe-
veral Lengths and Bores.
3. *A Glafs-Tunnel or two, with wooden difhes and fpoons, for*
filling of the Glafs-Tubes with Mercury.
4. *You muft have no Metalline Utenfils about you, for fear they*
be fpoiled with the Mercury.
5. *Spread a Blanket or Carpet on the ground when you try thefe*
Experiments, that fo none of the Mercury *may be loft,*
but may be taken up again with wooden fpoons.
6. *You may have by you alfo Glafs-Syphons, Weather-Glaffes*
of feveral right and crooked fhapes, &c. the more to ad-
vantage the Experiments.

Figure 7.3 Page 88 of *Experimental Philosophy* listing requirements
for the mercury experiments

Henry Power's mercury experiments

Book 2 of *Experimental Philosophy* describes Power's experiments with mercury,
which commenced in Cambridge and continued at his home, Elland Hall near
Halifax.[44] He first describes the apparatus required (p. 88), (Figure 7.3) then many
experiments. Using tubes of eight lengths the quicksilver 'will descend in tubes of
greater length than 29 inches' and 'will not descend lower than 29 inches',
irrespective of tube length and diameter (p. 90). Adding mercury to the vessel
causes the mercury level to rise and 'contrariwise, if you take any Quicksilver out
of the vessel, that in the tube decends lower'(p. 91). And, 'if you tilt or incline the
Glass-Tube, you shall see the Quicksilver gradually to ascend'. And, 'If you

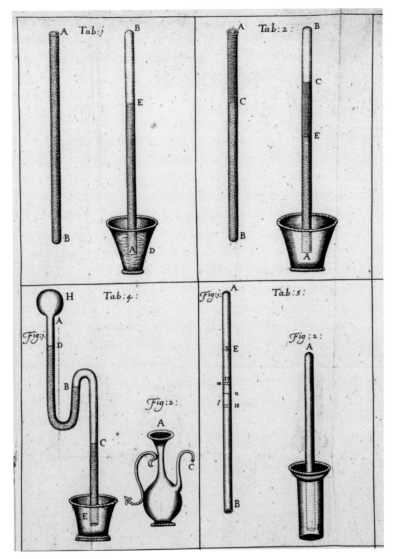

Figure 7.4 Four drawings selected from nine, illustrating various mercury experiments.

immerge the Tube into Vessels of Quicksilver of several capacities and larger Surfaces, the descent of it will not alter.' (p. 93). Then follow experiments with the vacuum, introducing air and water, and observing how the collapsed swim bladder of a fish expands. Figure 7.4 illustrates four of the nine drawings of these experiments. The description of a mercury 'altimeter' begins in 'Experiment 7', the quotation from which begins this article. The manuscript account is illustrated. Power considered that his mercury column would 'Mechanically find out the Perpendicular height of our great Hill [775 feet] here at Halifax', and wished that 'some of our Canary-Merchants would get this Experiment try'd at the top of the Pike of Teneriffe, which is deservedly famed for the highest Hill in the world'.

Power's experimental work lessened as his practice as a physician expanded after gaining his MD in 1655. He was also occupied by extensive alterations to his house, New Hall.[45] A few years later he resumed his experiments with Richard Townley of Townley Hall, Lancashire.[46]

SUMMARY AND CONCLUSIONS

The discovery of the barometer in France, Italy and England has been traced. The vertical limit of the suction pump was observed by Beeckman in Caen, and that of the syphon by Baliani in Genoa. *Via* Galileo, the idea of a column of water supported by air pressure – disbelieved by Galileo – came to a group of scientists in Rome, including Berti from Mantua, and Torricelli from Florence. Berti in Rome made the critical experiment that a column of water of 18 cubits could be supported by air pressure, and Torricelli, home in Florence, with the assistance of his colleague Viviani, performed the first experiment using mercury, the modest height of the column being that postulated by Viviani and suggested by Galileo. The 'Torricellian experiment', with many variations, was commonly performed in France and England, principally through the connections of Mersenne in Paris. To Pascal, in Paris, came the idea that the height of the mercury column would vary with altitude, and this was demonstrated by his brother-in-law, Perier, in an ascent of the *Puy-de-Dome* in Auvergne and published in Paris by the anatomist Pecquet. The reading of Pecquet's book gave Power the idea of the mercury level varying with altitude and prompted many new variations of the 'Torricellean Experiment'.

Finally, we carry the story forward a few years. The Royal Society was formed in 1660 and Power became a member through John Tillotson (1630-1694), a boyhood friend from Halifax and a future Archbishop of Canterbury.[47] His admission was proposed on 8 May 1661 and earlier that year, the Society, had adopted Power's suggestion of Mount Teide, Teneriffe and resolved to 'Try the Quicksilver experiment at the top, and several other ascents of the mountain'.[48] Power performed more experiments in collaboration with Richard Townley in Lancashire, ascending Pendle Hill near Townley.[49] 'Subterraneous Experiments or Observations about Cole-Mines' took his mercury columns below ground.[50] These were reported to scientists in London and to Boyle and Hooke in Oxford, and from them arose the idea of air pressure being related to volume – Boyle's Law.

Power had in 1666 removed to Wakefield with his wife, his daughter Ellen, and his son George – Jane his second daughter died young. Power died 23 December 1668 and was buried in the Parish Church, Wakefield, where a large brass plate attests his local fame.[51]

ACKNOWLEDGEMENTS

I am indebted to the staffs of the Bodleian, Cambridge, British, and Halifax Libraries. Geoffrey Martin (Christ's College) and Jacqueline Cox (Cambridge University Archives) kindly checked entries of Power. I thank the British Library for permission to reproduce figure 4 from BL *Sloane 1393, ff. 144.*

NOTES AND REFERENCES

1 Power H, *Experimental Philosophy, in Three Books: Containing New Experiments, Microscopical, Mercurial, Magnetical.* (1663) (hereafter Power, *Experimental Philosophy*). [Power's copy in the British Library is dated 1663 in his handwriting].

2 But less explicitly than Boyle. Boyle's publication date was 1662. But White Kennet in *Register and Chronicle*, 1728, 541, records a second book by Power, published in September 1661. This was book 2 of *Experimental Philosophy*.

3 Accounts of Power's life are in: Peile J, *Biographical Register of Christ's College*, 2 vols. Cambridge: 1910, vol. 1, 477; Clay J.W, 'Dr Henry Power of New Hall, F.R.S.', *Transactions of the Halifax Antiquarian Society*, [These transactions had no volume number] (1917), 1-31; Pedigree in Ralph Thoresby's *Ducatus Leodiensis*, ed. T.D. Whitaker 1816, 258; *Dictionary of National Biography*. Oxford: 1998, (hereafter *DNB*), vol. 16, 256.

4 Thoresby, *Ducatus Leodiensis*, 258.

5 C. Giles, 'New Hall, Elland; The Story of a Pennine Gentry House from c. 1490 to the mid-19th Century'. In *Old West Riding*. Oldgate, Huddersfield: 1981, ed. G. Redmonds. Vol. 1. No. 2.

6 Hughes J.T, 'Sir Thomas Browne, Shibden Dale, and the Writing of *Religio Medici*.', *Yorkshire History Quarterly*, Settle, 5 (2000), 89-94.

7 His memorial plaque in Wakefield Parish Church records his death in 1668 at the age of forty-five years, making his birth in 1623. The register of Christ's College, Cambridge gives his age on 9 June 1641 as fifteen years, giving a birth date of 1626.

8 Venn J, and Venn J.A, *Alumni Cantabridgienses*. Cambridge: 1924: part 1, vol. 3, 389. Pensioners were sons of clergy or small land owners.

9 Barwick J, *Querela Cantabrigensis*. Oxford: 1646, 10-11.

10 de Waard C, *L'experience barometrique, ses antecedents et ses explications. Etude historique.* Thouars, 1936; Knowles Middleton W.E, 'The Place of Torricelli in the History of the Barometer', *Isis, Philadelphia*, 54 (1963), 11-28.

11 Webster C, 'The Discovery of Boyle's Law, and the Concept of the Elasticity of Air in the Seventeenth Century', *Archive for History of Exact Sciences*, 2 (1965), 441-502.

12 Galileo G, *Le Opera*. Florence: 1894, IV, 167.

13 Beeckman came from the Low Countries: what is now Belgium.

14 Beeckman I, *MD thesis, University of Caen*. An incomplete copy survives in the British Library, *BL. 1179. d.9 (3)*.

15 *Journal tenu par lui de 1604 a 1634, publie avec une introduction et des notes par Cornelius de Waard*. 4 Vols. Paris: La Haye, 1939-1953. The quotation is from 1, 36.

16 de Waard C, *Correspondence de P. Marin Mersenne, religieux minime*. vols. 1-17. Paris: 1936, 2, 282-283.

[17] Rey J, *Essai sur la recherche de la cause pour laquelle l'estain et la plomb augmentent de poids quand on les calcine*. Bazas, 1630.

[18] Galileo G, *Le Opera*, XIV. 1904 127-130.

[19] Galileo G, *Dialogues concerning two new sciences*. English translation of the 1638 text by H. Crew and A. de Salvio. London and New York: 1914. Reprint New York: 1954.

[20] The correspondence appears in *Le Opera*, XIV (1904), 124-125 and 159.

[21] Gaspar Berti does not appear in the *Italian Biographical Index*, Munich, 1993, which combines entries from 321 Italian biographical reference works.

[22] Maignan E, *Cursus philosophicus concinnatus ex notissimis cuique principis*. Toulouse: 1653. The four volumes are paged as one, 1925-1936.

[23] In the *Vienna Nationalbibliothek MS. 7049, letter CXXVII*. The Italian text is given in *de Waard*, 178-181.

[24] de Waard, *L'experience barometrique*, 180.

[25] Knowles Middleton, *Isis*, 11-28.

[26] The page of Galileo's manuscript is reproduced in Knowles Middleton, p. 18.

[27] Knowles Middleton, 19.

[28] Torricelli's two letters to Ricci are reproduced (translated) in Knowles Middleton, 19-24.

[29] Knowles Middleton, *Isis*, 27.

[30] de Waard, *L'experience barometrique*, 119.

[31] Appears in *Oeuvres de Plaise Pascal*, ed. L. Brunschicg and P. Boutroux. Paris: 1908, 2, 365-373.

[32] Pecquet J, *Experimenta nova anatomica*. Paris: 1651.

[33] Georgi Sinclari, *Ars Nova et Magna Gravitas et Levitas*. Roterodami: 1669, *Dialogus Primus*, 125-149.

[34] For the knowledge in England of the work in Paris see Webster, 1965, 454-458.

[35] Sheffield University Library, *Hartlib papers Bundle VII, no. 29*. The letter is reproduced in Webster, 1965, 456.

[36] Roach J.R.C, *A History of the County of Cambridge, and the Isle of Ely*. 1959.

[37] The Regius Chair of Physic was created by Henry VIII in 1540. The earlier Linacre Lectureship in Physic was established at St. John's College in 1524.

[38] Walker R.M, 'Francis Glisson', in A. Rook, ed., *Cambridge and its Contribution to Medicine*. London: Wellcome Institute of the History of Medicine, 1971, 35-47.

[39] Browne T, *The Works of Sir Thomas Browne*, vols, 1-6, G. Keynes, ed. 1928-31, The correspondence of Power and Browne appears in vol. 6, 275-295.

[40] Browne, *Works*, 6, 277-278.

[41] Browne, *Works*, 6, 282-283.

[42] See *DNB* for biographies of Whichcote, 21, pp. 1-3; More, 13, 868-870; Cudworth, 5, 271-275; and Smith, 18, 482-483.

[43] British Library, *Sloane MS, 1333 ff. 133-141*, and *Sloane MS 1393, ff. 134-153*; and Bodleian Library, *Ashmolean MS 1400, ff. 15-21*.

[44] Power, *Experimental Philosophy*, 85-149.

[45] Stead J, Dr Henry Power and his alterations at New Hall, Elland. In *Old West Riding Books*, ed. J. Stead. Huddersfield: 1980, vol 8, 8-17.

46 Webster C, 'Richard Towneley (1629-1707), The Townley Group and Seventeenth-Century Science', *Transactions of the Historic Society of Lancashire and Cheshire*, 118 (1966), 51-76.

47 *DNB*, 19, 872-878.

48 Birch T, *History of the Royal Society of London*, 4 vols. 1756-7, 1, 22 and 8.

49 Power, *Experimental Philosophy*, 121-137.

50 Power, *Experimental Philosophy*, 171-181.

51 Thomas Gent of York, *The Ancient and Modern History of the Loyal Town of Ripon*. York 1673-1778, 13-73.

Dr Henry Power (1626-1668):
The Medical Practice of a Halifax Physician

> Sacred to the memory of Henry Power, Doctor of Medicine, whose loss is universally regretted, who had a clear head, a sound judgement, together with all the accomplishments of a good Christian and a fine gentleman. And, had he lived longer, those great masters Hippocrates and Aesculapius might not only have been his pupils in their own profession, but in most other branches of polite and useful learning.

The text above translates part of the Latin on a brass plate in the floor of the middle chancel near the altar of the church of All Saints, Wakefield, where Henry Power was buried on December 23rd 1668.[1] [2] Dr Henry Power is known, not only as a physician, but as a scientist, and a founder of the Royal Society.[3] This article describes his medical practice, mainly from New Hall, Elland, Halifax.[4] Power's papers in the British Library include the financial accounts of his practice in Halifax.[5]

The Power Family

Henry's father, John Power – described as the 'Spanish Merchant' – was in trade, in contrast to the elder sons of the Power family, who, after Cambridge, became clergymen. John was the youngest of the four sons of William Power, Rector of Barwick in Elmet, and there were two daughters. One daughter, Ann, married the Rev. John Favour, Vicar of Halifax, a connection that brought her brother, John, to Halifax, where he became a large property owner. He married Jane, daughter of a Mr Jennings, possibly from Erdington, near Birmingham. They had a daughter, Ellen, and four sons, our subject, Henry, then John, Thomas, and William. John remained in Halifax whilst Ellen, Thomas, and William migrated to London.[6]

Birth and Schooling

John and Jane Power lived for a time in Annesley, Notts, where John probably had business with the family of Sir George (later Viscount) Chaworth, whose country seat was Annesley Hall.[7] [8] [9]

Richard Hall engraved a picture of Annesley Hall (Figure 8.1) *circa* 1677.[10] No baptismal record for Henry has been found but 'Ellen Power daughter of John Power gent, baptised 7 June 1624' appears in the register of baptisms for Annesley Church, now a ruin.[11] The development of the smelting of iron and lead, and later of coal mining expanded the population and in 1874, a new church, All Saints, replaced the old to serve what was now a colliery village. Henry was probably

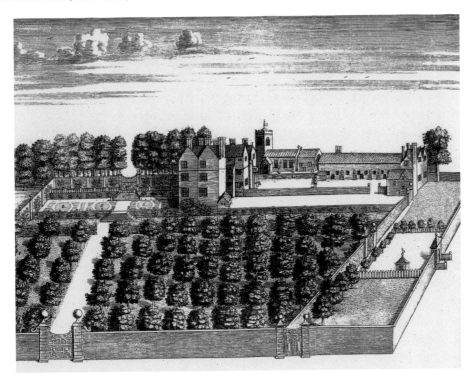

Figure 8.1 The South East prospect of Annesley House, as seen from the Park Gate, Nottingham Road, and engraved by Richard Hall.
In R. Thornton: *The Antiquities of Nottinghamshire*, (Nottingham, 1677), facing p. 252.

born at Annesley in 1626.[12] The family moved to Halifax, possibly about 1633, the date that John Power purchased the Multure Hall.

Which school Henry attended is uncertain. Cambridge records state 'Halifax under Higginson', but accounts of the Heath Grammar School at Woodhouse, Halifax, do not mention Power or Higginson.[13] Some Halifax boys boarded at York.[14] An important childhood experience was meeting Sir Thomas Browne, then a young doctor, fresh from continental education, residing in Halifax, and composing his renowned *'Religio Medici'*.[15] Browne had probably met John Power on the Continent, which connection brought Browne to Halifax. Henry, about twelve years old, was influenced by Browne, and directed into a career in medicine. John Power died in 1638 and Henry's mother swiftly remarried, her new husband being Anthony Foxcroft, who owned New Hall, Elland, to which the family moved. But the subsequent ownership of New Hall is complex – see below.

Cambridge University

Power was fifteen years old when he matriculated at Cambridge University on 9 June, 1641 as a pensioner of Christ's College under the care of Mr Wilding.[16] Christ's was the preferred College of the Power family, and Henry's uncle, William, was then a Fellow of the College, and the Lady Margaret Preacher.[17] Henry spent 14 profitable years at Cambridge, the first three studying classics for his BA, awarded in 1644/5.[18] His MA followed in 1648. Lectures and seminars occupied the three terms, and, importantly, dinners were taken in College, when students shared the company of the fellows. During vacations Henry returned to Halifax. In 1645, after his BA, Henry began medical studies towards his MD, omitting a BM degree, which omission was then possible in Cambridge. Christ's College, with several medical fellows, was prominent in medicine – as were St John's, Emmanuel, and Caius –, but was also the college of the 'Cambridge Platonists', who viewed Christianity as a continuation of Platonic ideals.[19] [20] Notable Platonists were Henry Moore, at Christ's from his entry in 1631 to his death in 1687, and Ralph Cudworth, formerly Master of Clare, but Master of Christ's from 1654.[21] The Cambridge Platonists, in particular Henry More, were important in introducing the ideas and discoveries of Descartes to England.[22] Power was at Christ's under two masters, Thomas Bainbridge, Master from 1622-1646, and Samuel Bolton, Master from 1646-1654.[23]

The Regius Professor of Physic was Francis Glisson, a famous physician, but also a physiologist and anatomist, now remembered for his *Anatomia hepatis*, published in 1654.[24] Influencing Cambridge from the Continent were publications in medicine and science, of which subjects Power wrote to Dr Browne:

> Sr, I have now by the frequency of living & dead dissections of Doggs, run through the whole body of Anatomy Insisting on Spigelius, Bartholinus, Fernelius, Columbus, Veslingius, but especially Harvey's Circulation, & the two Incomparable Authors, Descartes, & Regius[25]

Power's studies were enlarged by a comprehensive library, modelled on that of Browne.[26] Power's period in Cambridge (1641-1655) spanned the Civil Wars (1642-1646 and 1648), the execution of the King (January, 1649), and the creation of the Protectorate.[27] The colleges of Cambridge were purged by the Earl of Manchester – Commander of the Parliamentary forces – who in March 1643/4 removed nine Masters from the headship of their colleges. At Christ's, Thomas Bainbridge was allowed to remain, but nine fellows were ejected, amongst them William Power, Henry's uncle. The disruption to the College is evident by the numbers of admissions, 27 in 1641-1642, but 15 in 1642-1643, and only 12 in 1643-1644. In 1644-1645 numbers had returned to 58, and in 1645-1646, there were 52 admissions.[28]

Return to Halifax

Power began his medical practice in Halifax *circa* 1652, but already in 1649 he was writing from Halifax to Dr Browne '...to give me some Practicall method of the cure of some common diseases...'[29] Strictly he required his Cambridge MD, which was conferred in 1655, but regulations, preventing his medical practice in

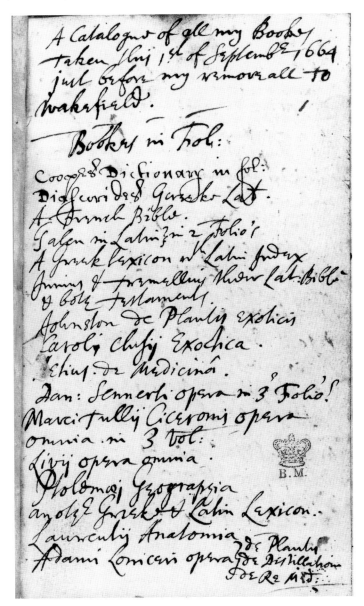

Figure 8.4 First page of Henry Power's 'Catalogue of all my Books', dated 1 September, 1964. Reproduced, by permission of the British Library, from *Sloane MS. 1346*.

bleeding and blistering, the use of which persisted for many years, being cruelly applied to Charles II, accelerating his death in 1685.

Power did not use bleeding or blistering, nor did he prescribe emetics, and his purgatives were probably mild laxatives. He was interested in chemistry and might have taken up the ideas of the Paracelsians, had these been more accessible to him.[43] His therapies were medicinal herbs, which he grew in his garden, gathered in the fields, or procured from suppliers. His library had many herbal textbooks.

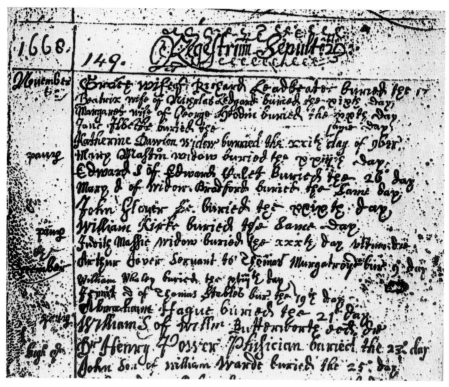

Figure 8.5 Entry of Power's burial at Wakefield on 23 December, 1668. Reproduced, by permission from the registrar in Library Headquarters, Wakefield, west Yorkshire.

Closing Years at Wakefield

We can only conjecture why in 1664, Power, from living in a house much altered to his liking, should move to Wakefield. Clay suggests:

> having got good customers among the surrounding gentry, who, perhaps, were more numerous than in the Halifax district, it would be more convenient for him.[44]

His Memorandum Book notes his move: '... that I came to Wakefield to live 7 of October 1664 wch was on a Friday.'[45] After this date, the entries of visits, prescriptions, and fees continue but are more directed to patients around Wakefield. And accounts of repairs and alterations switch to his house in Wakefield, which, it seems, from hearth taxes, was large, a parsonage with eight hearths.[46]

There is evidence in his letters that he was now in poor health, which might explain his move to Wakefield, a more gentle area than the robust Calderdale valley. His lucrative practice continued but his scientific experiments ceased, as did his researches into botany and zoology. He died in 1668 (Figure 8.5), and was buried on 23 December, in All Saints, Wakefield Parish Church, now the

Cathedral. His will, drawn up on 19 December, 1668, was proved on 2 June, 1669, by his widow.[47]

Margery remained in the house in Wakefield for a further eight years, returning to Halifax on 6 December, 1676.[48] Her son, George, now sixteen, inherited New Hall, when he came of age. There is evidence that he entered in 1681, with a child and a lady who was not his wife. George lived an irregular and unremunerative life, and died in 1700, unmarried, and with no legal heirs. John Hanson of Backall, Southowram, inherited New Hall, which then suffered a decline, through several owners, but survived to be restored in the present century. It is now a private residence.

With the death of George, the line of Henry Power was extinguished, further obscuring the memory of Power. But his memorial plaque, in what is now Wakefield Cathedral, reminds us of a great physician and scientist, who practiced in Halifax and Wakefield.

ACKNOWLEDGEMENTS

I am indebted to the staffs of the Bodleian, Cambridge, British, and Halifax Libraries, to Adrian Henstock, Archivist in Nottingham, for figure 8.1, and to Mrs D Scriven, Archivist in Wakefield, for figure 8.5. Figures 8.2 and 8.3 are reproduced from photographs BB68/9028 and BB68/9047 of the National Monument Record, Swindon. I thank the British Library for permission to reproduce figure 8.4 from BL *Sloane 1346.f.1*

NOTES AND REFERENCES

[1] Thomas Gent of York, *The Ancient and Modern History of the Loyal Town of Rippon.* York: 1763, 13 - 14.

[2] Sisson J.L, *Historic Sketch of the Parish Church, Wakefield.* Wakefield: 1824, 40-41.

[3] Accounts of Henry Power are in: Ralph Thoresby's *Ducatus Leodiensis*, ed. T.D. Whittaker: 1816, 258; Peile J, *Biographical Register of Christ's College*, 2 vols. Cambridge: 1910, vol 1, 477; Clay J.W, 'Dr Henry Power of New Hall, F.R.S.', *Transactions of the Halifax Antiquarian Society* (henceforth *THAS*), Halifax, (1917), 1-31; Venn J. and Venn J.A, *Alumni Cantabrigiensis*. Cambridge: 1924, part 1, vol 3, 389; *Dictionary of National Biography*. Oxford: 1998, vol 16, 256.

[4] The house is described in: Giles C, 'New Hall, Elland; the story of a Pennine Gentry House from *c.* 1490 to the mid-19th Century', *Old West Riding*, vol. 1, no. 2, Ed. Geo Redmonds. Oldgate, Huddersfield: 1981, 1-11; and Stead J, 'Dr Henry Power and his Alterations at New Hall Elland 1655-1664', *Old West Riding*, vol. 8, no. 2, Ed. Stead J. Oldgate, Huddersfield: 1988, 8-17.

[5] British Library, *Memorandum Books, 7 vols. Sloane MSS.1351, 1353-1358.*

[6] Thomas became a stationer, William a haberdasher, and Ellen married a William Howson, *Clay*, p.31.

[7] Throsby J, *History of Nottinghamshire*. Nottingham: 1790, vol. 2, 266-270.

[8] I am indebted to Adrian Henstock, Archivist in Nottingham, for information about Annesley.

[9] A deed of 1633 describes John Power as late of Arnold, Nottinghamshire, and now of Halifax. Hanson J.W, 'The Multure Hall', *TWAS*, (1935), 1-19.

[10] In Robert Thoroton, *The Antiquities of Nottinghamshire*. Nottingham: 1677, facing p. 252.

[11] Nottinghamshire Archives, *Register of baptisms for Annesley, 1624-1633, PR 2826*.

[12] Cambridge records. *Peile*, 1910, 477 and *Venn & Venn* 389. On entering Christ's College, Henry was 15, and his birthplace was given as Annesley, Notts.

[13] Cox T, *A Popular History of the Grammar School of Queen Elizabeth at Heath, Halifax*. Halifax: 1879.

[14] Stead, p. 8.

[15] Hughes J.T, 'Sir Thomas Browne, Shibden Dale, and the Writing of Religio Medici', *Yorkshire History Quarterly*, 5, (2000) 89-94.

[16] Pensioners were sons of clergy or small landowners. Above them were fellow-commoners, sons of aristocrats: below them were sizars, the poor students.

[17] For the history of the College see: Peile J, *Christ's College*. London: 1900.

[18] Peile, 1910, 1, 477.

[19] Peile, 1900, 176-206.

[20] Patrides C.A, *The Cambridge Platonists*. London: 1969, and Cambridge: 1980.

[21] Pawson G.P.H, *The Cambridge Platonists and their Place in Religious Thought*. London: 1930.

[22] M. Nicholson, 'The Early Stage of Cartesianism in England', *Studies in Philology*: 26 (1929), 356-374.

[23] Peile, 1900, 165.

[24] Rolleston H.D, *The Cambridge Medical School*. Cambridge: 1932, 151-155.

[25] Letter to Dr Browne, 15 September, 1648. British Library, *MS. Sloane 1911-1913, f.80*. In Keynes G, *The Works of Sir Thomas Browne*, vols 1-6. London: Faber and Gwyer, becoming Faber and Faber. 1928-31, 6, 283.

[26] Catalogue of 'all my books' before Power's move from Halifax to Wakefield in 1664. British Library, *Sloane MS. 1346*.

[27] Peile, 1900, 160-175.

[28] Peile, 1900, 165.

[29] Letter to Browne, August 28th, 1649, *MS. Sloane 1911-1913, f. 82*. Reproduced in Keynes, 6, 287-288.

[30] Hughes J.T, Henry Power (1626-1668) of New Hall, Elland and Experiments on Barometric Pressure, *THAS*, (2002), 14-26.

[31] The sequence of building was researched by Giles, 1-11.

[32] Described by Stead, 8-17.

[33] Webster C, 'Richard Towneley (1629-1707), the Towneley Group and Seventeenth-Century Science', *Transactions of the Historic Society of Lancashire and Cheshire*, Liverpool, 118 (1966), 51-76.

[34] British Library, *Sloane MSS. 1351 ff. 1-144, 1353 ff. 1-124, 1354 ff. 1-96, 1355 ff. 1-72, 1356 ff. 1-111, 1357 ff. 1-120, 1358 ff. 1-69*.

[35] Clay, *THAS*, 1-31.

[36] Midgely S, *Hallifax and its Gibbet-Law Placed in a True Light*, printed by J. How for William Bentley. Halifax: 1708.

[37] A Jonathan Maud, of Halifax, was created MD in June, 1652, because '... he hath been a constant friend to the parliament...' Anthony A Wood, *Athenae Oxoniensis & The Fasti*, ed. P Bliss. London, 1820, vol. 4, 173.

[38] Raach J.H, *A Directory of English Country Physicians 1603-1643*. London: 1962, 119-128.

[39] Goods were transported by pack animals traversing a narrow paved path called a 'causey'. Clegg C, 'Coaching Days', *THAS*, (1923), 123-158.

[40] 'A catalogue of all my Books taken the 1st of September 1664 just before my removall to Wakefield', *Sloane MS. 1346*.

[41] Temkin O, *Galenism: Rise and Decline of a Medical Philosophy*. Ithaca and London: 1973, 103.

[42] Simples, made from one species of herb, affected one humour. Compounds, from two or more herbs, had a main effect and a second effect. Entities were 'efficient' drugs, which included purgatives, emetics, poisons, and antidotes, and had one specific action but on the whole body.

[43] See Debus A.G, *The English Paracelsians*. New York: 1966.

[44] Clay, 6.

[45] *Sloane, MS 1358 f. 1.*

[46] Stead, p. 13, note 19.

Observations and Experiments of Dr Henry Power (1626-1668) supporting William Harvey's *De Motu Cordis*

> There has not one Day pass'd, since that worthy production of his was first deliver'd into the world, but it hath mett with men of sevral humours and constitutions, some with very smart and active Discourse maintaining and avouching it, others with as much vehemency and passion busily refuting it... Amongst all the rabble of his antagonists, wee see not one that attempts to fight him at his own weapon, that is by sensible and Anatomical evictions to Confute that, which hee has by Sense and Autopsy so vigourously Confirm'd.[1]

Henry Power (1626-1668) of Halifax, scientist and physician, is best known for his many experiments.[2] His medical practice in Halifax was also extensive.[3] He was a founder member of the Royal Society of London but his work in Yorkshire attracted less attention than contemporary research in Oxford, Cambridge, and London. He died young, having published only one book, which however establishes his scientific eminence.[4] His work on air pressure preceded and influenced that of Robert Boyle (1627-1691)[5] His microscopical observations were published before those of Robert Hooke (1635-1703).[6] Power left many manuscripts, now in the British and Bodleian libraries.[7] The quotation above is from his extensive notes under the heading *Circulatio Sanguinis, Inventio Harveiana*, dated 1652, the subject of this article.

Power and Harvey

Henry Power, of a family centred on Halifax, was educated at Christ's College, Cambridge, entering in 1641.[8] He was directed into medicine by Sir Thomas Browne, who became a lifelong friend and confidant.[9] Browne guided Power in the Greek and Latin texts in science and medicine, but tutor and pupil were aware of contemporary writing in these subjects, also well known in Cambridge.[10] On 15 September 1648 Power writing to Browne reports that he had :

> ...run through the whole body of Anatomy Insisting on Spigelius, Bartholinus, Fernelius, Columbus, Veslingius, but especially Harvey's Circulation, & the two Incomparable Authors, DesCartes, & Regius...[11]

Power, more than Browne, looked to recent and contemporary authors for guidance in science and medicine. He also extended and replicated observations and experiments, as in his work on the mercury barometer in 1653.[12] In anatomy, a year earlier, after studying the writings of Harvey on the circulation of the blood, he began a series of observations and experiments to confirm Harvey's work. In 1652 Power commenced his medical practice in Halifax, where his anatomical work, begun in Cambridge, was completed.[13]

Harvey and *De Motu Cordis*

The publication in 1628 by William Harvey (1578-1657) (Figure 9.1) on the circulation of the blood is a milestone in anatomy, physiology and medicine, possibly the greatest in the history of these subjects.[14] This was celebrated 300 years later.[15] There have been several modern translations.[16] These have been listed and discussed by K.J. Franklin.[17] The content of this book marks the transition between medicine and science based mainly on Aristotle and Galen, and modern observations and research, which today continue the work and teaching of Harvey, whose life has attracted many biographers.[18]

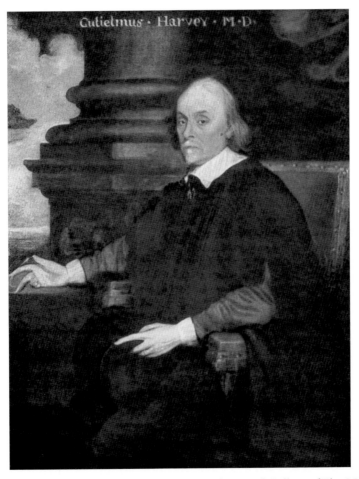

Figure 9.1. The portrait of William Harvey in the Royal College of Physicians, painted *circa* 1650. This figure and figs. 2, 3, & 6 are reproduced from Chauncey D. Leake (1941). Author's collection.

The profound change in thinking after 1628 is evident by comparison with the writings of Galen on the functions of the organs of body.[19] Galen viewed the organs as a system in which nutrients were assimilated and life force created. The food, after digestion in the stomach, became chyle, which passed through the portal vein into the liver to form blood. The blood entered the *vena cavae* and was distributed throughout the body by the veins. Part went to the right ventricle of the heart and, through the pulmonary arteries, nourished the lungs and was purified by the air. Some of the blood in the right ventricle went though pores into the left ventricle, and received air, or pneuma, from the trachea *via* the pulmonary vein. This air, containing vital spirit, acted on the blood in the left ventricle to form arterial blood, which passed with air into the aorta and all the arteries, including those to the brain.[20] There was an idea of ebb and flow of blood, but it was thought that most of the blood created in the liver was consumed in the tissues throughout the body. Galen's teaching of anatomy and physiology dominated understanding of disease, and prejudiced therapy, an example being the practice of bleeding to correct imbalance of body humours, when the side and place from where blood was removed was all important. Galen's teaching, inconsistent with modern anatomy and physiology, was the basis of medicine in Europe and the Arab world for over 1500 years.[21] There is a paradox in this enthusiasm for Aristotle and Galen. Medical teaching in Greek and Latin was largely lost in Europe – but not in the Arab world – during the dark ages, and was only regained in the sixteenth century, in England, due to Thomas Linacre (1460 ?– 1524) and John Caius (1510-1573).

The renaissance in sixteenth century Europe, most active in Italy, revised anatomy and physiology, although the church was reluctant to sanction departures from ancient texts, which, in medicine, were those of Aristotle and Galen.[22] Modern anatomy benefited from the practice of anatomical dissection, and permanent anatomy theatres were erected, the first, at Padua, in 1594, by Fabricius.[23] Animal experiments began the modern study of physiology.[24] The University of Padua was protected by nearby Venice, a wealthy and powerful city, usually independent of Rome. The tolerance of Padua in admitting protestants attracted many foreign medical students, one of whom was Harvey (Figure 9.1), who came in 1600, and obtained his medical degree in 1602. Fabricius, who taught Harvey, had published *De venarum ostiolis* in 1603.[25] The deduction by Harvey that these valves in the veins permitted blood flow only in one direction – towards the heart – led Harvey to his discovery of the circulation.[26]

Forerunners of Harvey

De Motu Cordis was the fruit of years of observations and experiments, many of which Harvey described in his annual Lumleian lectures (Figure 9.2).[27] But ancient and more recent researchers had made significant contributions.[28] Erasistratus

(330-245 B.C.) had traced the veins and arteries to the heart and described the auriculo-ventricular valves, but believed the arteries contained air.[29] Aristotle (384-322 B.C.) and Galen (131-200 A.D.) knew the arteries contained blood, but whilst Aristotle believed the heart was central to the supply of blood, Erasistratus and Galen thought that the liver continuously created blood.

The pulmonary circulation had been described in the thirteenth century by Ibn Nafis, a physician in Cairo, and a translation into Latin may have existed in the sixteenth century.[30] This lesser circulation was also described by Servetus, who wrote: 'By a signal artifice ...the subtle blood is driven through the lungs and cleansed from its fumes, so at length it is stuff fit to become the vital spirit'.[31] For this and other heresies, Servetus was burnt alive in Geneva, in 1553, with nearly all the thousand copies of his offending book, *Restitutio Christianismi*.[32]

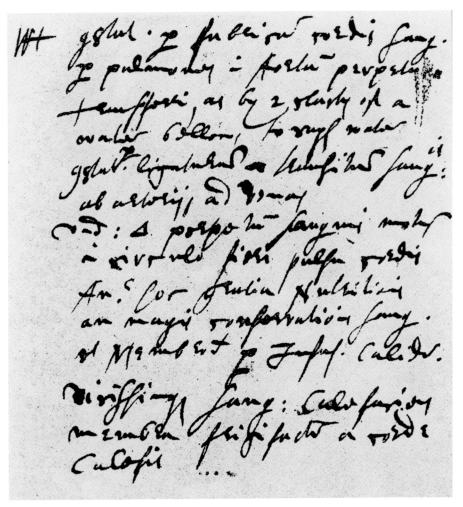

Figure 9.2. Harvey's first description of the circulation of the blood on p. 80 of his 1616 lecture notes. The Latin is in Harvey's hand and his initials appear top left.

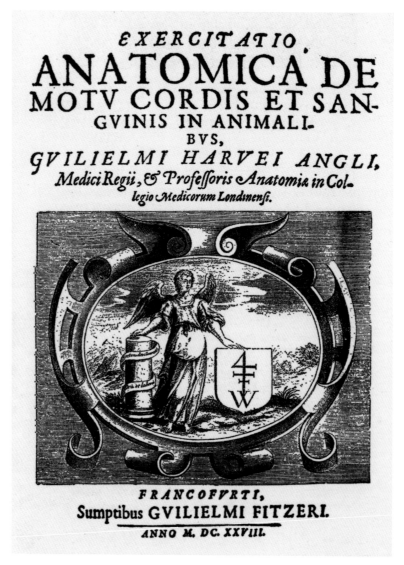

Figure 9.3. Title Page of the first edition (1628) of *De Motu Cordis*.

The modern anatomical concepts of Servetus have attracted much attention.[33] The pulmonary circulation was also known to Columbus (1516-1559) and Cesalpinus (1519-1603).[34] Servetus disproved Galen's statement that channels in the intraventricular septum permitted blood to pass between the ventricles, also doubted by Vesalius.[35] Nor could Leonardo da Vinci, who performed more than 100 autopsies, find Galen's pores.[36]

Supporters and Opponents of Harvey

De Motu Cordis was indifferently printed in Frankfurt with a small type face on paper of poor quality (Figure 9.3). There were numerous misprints due to difficult communications between author and printer: proofs were not sent and corrected.[37] But the science was revolutionary, and, at first, attracted more criticism than praise. In England, James Primrose was Harvey's main opponent, but defence came from Robert Fludd, George Ent, Kenelm Digby, Thomas Bartholin, and Nathaniel Highmore.[38] Ole Worm in Copenhagen[39], Caspar Hofmann in Nuremberg[40], and Jean Riolan in Paris[41] were critics, but these were displaced by more worthy scientists, such as Rene Decartes, Johann Vesling, Frans de le Boe (Sylvius), and Jan de Wale. It is to this latter group, who examined the evidence at first hand, that Henry Power belongs. His support in 1652, based on a complete reappraisal of Harvey's observations and experiments, was important and welcome.

Sloane MS 1343, *Circulatio Sanguinis, Inventio Harveiana*

The manuscript consists of some 150 pages bound as a book (14 x 9 cms), written, on both sides in English, in the hand of Power, whose signature often appears (Figure 9.4 & 9.5).[42] The notes are divided into chapters and subdivided into 'experiments'. An experiment might be an operation on a living animal, usually a dog, but more often is an observation on a human or animal necropsy. Some 'experiments' are statements of received opinion. It is not always possible to

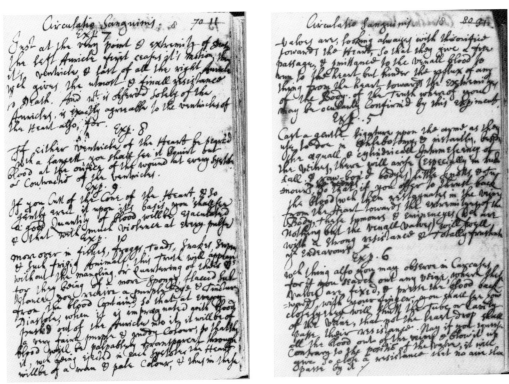

Figure 9.4 & 9.5. Pages of Power's manuscript, British Library, *Sloane MS 1343, ff. 8 & 18.*

determine whether Power is describing his own experiments and observations. Selections from the *MS* are described or quoted below:

Chapter 1. Explains how the laudable anatomical work of Aristotle and Galen has been extended, notably by 'our Reverend and Worthy Dr Harvey' who has 'the precedency for that Incomparable Invention of his, the Circulation of the Blood.' Anatomical studies are directed to areas hitherto obscure, but, above all, 'Living dissections ...by ocular Inspection to learn the abstrusity of hir [nature's] operations.'

Chapter 2. Describes opening the chest of a living animal and observing the 'Reciprocall motion and Quiescency which Anatomists call the contraction and Dilatation of the Heart.' In the slower heart beat of cold blooded animals such as amphibians, reptiles, and fishes the contraction and 'perisystole' [interval between systole and diastole] is more easily studied. In his interest in comparative anatomy, Power followed Harvey.[43] Power also describes the position and beat of the heart in the snail, louse, shrimp [probably Daphnia], crayfish, lobsters, crabs, and insects, but not in the bivalves (cockles, oysters and mussels), an error he shared with Harvey.[44]

Experiment 8. 'If either ventricle of the Heart be pearc'd .with a lancett, you shall see it squirt out blood ...at every systole or contraction of the ventricles'.

Experiment 12.
dissect a living dogge ...cutt of the left ventricle, so that the septum cordis or Partition-wall of the Heart, may be clearly visible, then observe if the right ventricle ayt every pulse sqeeze any blood through the septum, to be received by the left ventricle, according to the conceits and conjectural whimseys of the Ancients, which you shall find to be absolutely false.[45]

Experiment 14. Whilst the heart is in systole or contraction, all the arteries of the body pulse and are dilated.

Experiment 16. The pulse of all the arteries of the body is simultaneous, and is caused by the movement of the blood from the heart at systole.

Experiment 17. The pulse varies in frequency and vigour:
'Our experiencecomes closest to Cardan for wee have often tried by a minute-clock and found about 4000 pulses to passse in 1 hower'.

Experiment 18. A cut into the pulmonary artery causes an escape of blood when 'the Right ventricle shrinks into contraction'.

Experiment 19.
'Likewise if you Prick the Aorta, or any other artery ...you shall see the blood to jumpe out at every systole of the left ventricle...'

Experiment 21. From a transverse cut across the aorta of a dog, about half an ounce of blood is ejected at every pulse.

Experiment 22. Exsanguination of a dog by cutting the carotid artery yields about 3 gallons of blood.[46]

Experiment 27. If an artery is ligatured:

'you shall perceive a vehament intumescency twixt the ligature and the heart, but on the other side of the ligature a manfest Detumescency...'

Chapter 3. Of the veins and their valves.

Experiment 1.

'If you cast a ligature upon the vena cava, or any other veine... the Intumescency and Detumescency will appear just contrary to that in the Arteryes...'

Experiment 2. Occlude a vein near a man's wrist by manual pressure. With another hand, massage the blood in the vein towards the heart. If you release the second pressure, the vein does not refill, whilst it does when the first pressure is removed (Figure 9.6, from Harvey's *De Motu Cordis*).

Experiment 3. In phlebotomy following a ligature on the arm, bleeding is profuse when the vein is opened <u>below</u> the ligature. If the vein is lanced <u>above</u> the ligature it does not bleed.

Experiments 4-7. Details the valves of the veins. 6. In 'Carcases' when you press the vein with a finger the blood will only travel towards the heart. If you inflate with air a vein emptied of blood the air also will only proceed towards the heart.

Experiments 8 & 9. Valves are not present in arteries, except the beginnings of the pulmonary artery and the aorta.

Experiment 10. Power describes the ileocecal valve.

Experiment 11. Power describes a valve in the Eustacian tube, for which modern anatomists find no evidence.

Power then summarises his and Harvey's findings and description of the circulation. The contraction of left and right ventricles are simultaneous but the direction of the blood differs. From the right ventricle the blood passes to the lungs by the pulmonary artery, and by 'synastomoses or percribration through the spongy and porous substance of the lungs' enters the pulmonary veins and through the left auricle into the left ventricle. The contraction of the heart expels the blood into the aorta. The aortic valves prevent any retrograde flow and the blood 'is dispersed by the Branches, surcles and capillaryes of the Aorta, throughout every part of the body to be nourished.'

Power then turns to the:

only mystery to compleate this Circulatory motion, yet to be discovered is to explaine by what means the arteriall blood insuates itself into the veines and by

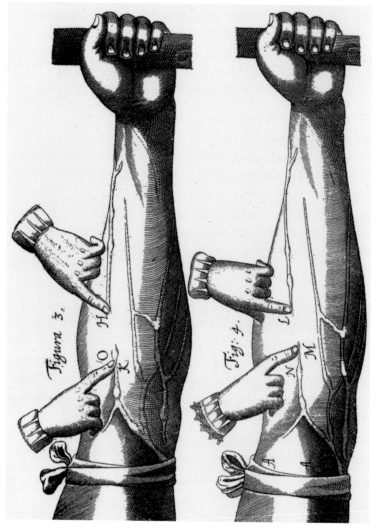

Figure 9.6. Figures 3 & 4 of *De Motu Cordis*, showing, with figures 1 & 2 (not illustrated),
how the valves regulate the filling of the veins.

what artifice and Contrivance in nature the Connection of these 2 Contrary
motions is performed.

In this passage, Power repeats the difficulty raised by Harvey and which was only
solved by the discovery of the capillaries by Malpighi in 1661. Power reviews
Harvey's estimates of the volume of blood in a person and the rapidity of its
circulation. The calculations are inaccurate by modern figures, but the importance
is that only a circulation of the blood would agree with the observations.

SUMMARY AND CONCLUSIONS

The publication, in 1628, of *De Motu Cordis*, by William Harvey is a turning point in medicine and biological sciences, when the outdated teaching of Aristotle and Galen began to be replaced by modern anatomy and physiology. The book, the fruit of many years of observations and experiments, established with certainty the circulation of the blood. The first reception was hostile, as the book overturned teaching held for hundreds of years, and backed by the authority of the church. Henry Power, completing his medical studies in Cambridge, confirmed the observations and experiments of Harvey, both in Cambridge, and at home in New Hall, Elland, near Halifax, Yorkshire. The British Library manuscript *Sloane MS 1343*, dated 1642, and the basis of this article, details the observations and experiments of Power confirming Harvey's discovery of the circulation of the blood. In England and in Europe many critics challenged the findings of Harvey. Of those who supported Harvey, importantly by repeating his work, a notable figure is Henry Power, whose work, described here, adds to his fame as a scientist and physician.

ACKNOWLEDGEMENTS

I am indebted to the staffs of the Bodleian, British, Cambridge, and Halifax libraries and the library of the Royal College of Physicians. Figures 9.4 & 9.5 are reproduced from *Sloane MS.1343*

NOTES AND REFERENCES

1 The manuscript notebook of Henry Power, *Circulatio sanguinis Inventio Harveiana*, British Library, *Sloane MS 1343*.

2 Hughes J.T, 'Henry Power (1626-1668) of New Hall, Elland and Experiments on Barometric Pressure', *Transactions of the Halifax Antiquarian Society*, 10, (2002), 14-26.

3 Hughes J.T, 'Dr Henry Power (1626-1668) : The Medical Practice of a Halifax Physician', *Transactions of the Halifax Antiquarian Society*, 11, (2003), 56-67.

4 Power H, *Experimental Philosophy, in Three Books : Containing New Experiments, Microscopical, Mercurial, Magnetical*. London: 1664. [Power's copy in the British Library is dated 1663 in his own handwriting.]

5 Webster C, 'The Discovery of Boyle's Law and the Concept of the Elasticity of Air in the Seventeenth Century', *Archive for the History of Exact Sciences*, 2, (1965), 441-502.

6 Although Power published in 1664 (or 1663, see note 4), Hooke's *Micrographia*, published in 1665, is a more comprehensive work on microscopy. Pierre Borel published his book *Centuria Observationum Microscopicarum*, in 1656. This book, now rare, was in Power's library.

[7] Most are in the British Library, *Sloane MSS*. The Bodleian Library has *Ashmolean MS 1400, ff. 15-21*.

[8] Matriculated 9 June, 1641, BA 1644/5, MA 1648, MD 1654/5.

[9] Hughes J.T, 'Sir Thomas Browne, Shibden Dale, and the Writing of *Religio Medici*.', *Yorkshire History Quarterly*, 5 (2000), Settle, Yorkshire, 89-94. Also Hughes (2003), 57.

[10] The correspondence between Power and Browne has been published by Keynes G, *The Works of Sir Thomas Browne*, vols 1-6. London: Faber and Gwyer, becoming Faber and Faber, 1928-1931, 6, 275-295.

[11] Keynes, 6, 293.

[12] Hughes, (2002).

[13] For a description and illustrations of his house, New Hall, Elland, Halifax see Hughes (2003).

[14] William Harvey. *Exercitatio Anatomica De Motu Cordis in Animalibus*. Frankfurt: William Fitzeri, 1628), usually abbreviated to *De Motu Cordis*. Fitzer was an English publisher in Frankfurt, suggested to Harvey by Robert Fludd. See Weil E, 'William Fitzer, the Publisher of Harvey's *De Motu Cordis*, 1628', *The Library*, 24, (1943), 142-164.

[15] In 1957, 300 years after Harvey's death, 'The William Harvey Issue' grouped articles in volume 12 of the *Journal of the History of Medicine and Allied Sciences* (henceforth *JHMAS*).

[16] Willis R, *The Works of William Harvey*. London: Sydenham Society, 1847; C.D. Leake, *Anatomical Studies on the Motion of the Heart and the Blood*, A modern English translation of William Harvey's *De Motu Cordis*. Springfield, Illinois, USA: Charles C. Thomas, 1928, 1931, & 1941; Franklin K.J, *Movement of the Heart and Blood in Animals*, by William Harvey, translated from the Latin. Oxford: Blackwell Scientific Publications, 1957; Whitteridge G, *An Anatomical Disputation Concerning the Movement of the Heart and Blood in Living Creatures*, by William Harvey, translated from the Latin. London: Blackwell Scientific Publications, 1976.

[17] The many translations of Harvey's works are described by Franklin K.J, 'On translating Harvey', *JHMAS*, 114-119.

[18] Chauvois L, Two editions, translated into French, *Vie de William Harvey* (Paris: Editions Sedes, 1957), and into English, *The Life of William Harvey*, London: Hutchinson, 1957; Power, D'Arcy, *William Harvey*. London: T. Fisher Unwin, 1897; Keynes G, *The Life of William Harvey*. Oxford: The Clarendon Press, 1978.

[19] Galen described the cardiovascular system in *On Anatomical Procedures*, Book VII, translated by C. Singer. London, Wellcome Foundation, 1956, 172-200, and in *De Usu Partium*, Books VI & VII.

[20] The latin *arteria* means windpipe.

[21] Wilfrid Bonser, 'General Medical practice in Anglo-Saxon England', In *Science, Medicine, and History*, two volumes, edited by E.A. Underwood. London: Oxford University Press, 1953, 1, 154-163.

[22] O'Malley C.D, 'Medical Education during the Renaissance', In *The History of Medical Education*, edited by C.D. O'Malley. Berkeley, Los Angeles & London: 1970, 89-102.

23 Girolamo Fabrizi d'Acquapendente, Professor of Anatomy during Harvey's medical studies at Padua.

24 For an analysis of Harvey's experiments see Macleod J.J.R, 'Harvey's experiments on circulation', *Annals of Medical History*, 10 (1928), 338-348.

25 Fabricius, *De venarum ostiolis*, (1603), edited by K.J. Franklin. Springfield, Illinois, 1933. Earlier anatomists had described the valves. See J.O. Leibowitz, 'Early accounts of the valves in the veins', *JHMAS*, 189-196.

26 Conversation of Harvey with Boyle. See Cohen H, 'The Germ of an idea or what put Harvey on the scent', *JHMAS*, 102-105; and Byleby J.J, 'Boyle and Harvey on the Valves in the Veins', *Bulletin of the History of Medicine*, 56, (1982), 351-367.

27 For a detailed account of Harvey's work see Bayon H.P, *Annals of Science*, (1938), Parts I & II, 3, pp. 59-118; (1938), Part 111, 3, pp. 435-456; and (1939), Part IV, 4, 65-106.

28 Rolleston H, 'Harvey's Predecessors and Contemporaries', *Annals of Medical History*, 10, (1928), 323-337.

29 Erasistratus of Ceos, founded the school of anatomy in Alexandria. Aristotle of Stagiri, was a pupil in Plato's academy in Athens, where he became a teacher. Galen, of Pergamon, studied in Smyrna, Corinth and Alexandria, and moved to Rome, where he practised as a physician.

30 Haddad Sami I. and Khairallah Amin A, 'A forgotten chapter in the history of the circulation of the blood', *Annals of Surgery*, 104, (1936), 1-8; O'Malley Charles D, 'A Latin translation of Ibn Nafis (1547) related to the problem of the circulation of the blood', *JHMAS*, 248-253.

31 Guthrie D, 'The Evolution of Cardiology', in *Science, Medicine, And History*, 2 volumes, edited by E.A. Underwood. London: Oxford University Press, 1953, 2, 508-517.

32 Three copies of *Restitutio Christianismi* survive, in Vienna, Paris, and Edinburgh.

33 Osler W, 'Michael Servetus', *Johns Hopkins Hospital Bulletin*, 21, (1910), 1-11; O'Malley C.D, *Michael Servetus (1511?-1553), A translation of his Geographical, Medical, and Astrological Writing*. Berkeley, Los Angeles, USA: University of California Press, 1953.

34 Mattheus Realdus Columbus of Cremona, was the pupil of Vesalius at Padua. Andreas Cesalpino of Arezzo, taught at Pisa and Rome.

35 Vesalius' reservations on septal pores were published in the second edition of *De Fabrica Humani Corporis*, (1555), Book VI. See O'Malley C.D, *Andreas Vesalius of Brussels*. Berkley, Los Angeles, and London: University of California Press, 1965, 280-281.

36 O'Malley C.D. and Saunders J.B. de C.M, *Leonardo da Vinci on the human body*. New York: Henry Schuman, 1952, pp. 216-217.

37 Communication between author and publisher was hampered by the Thirty Years War (1618-1648).

38 For the literature from 1628-1657 see Weil E, 'The Echo of Harvey's *De Motu Cordis* (1628)' *JHMAS*, 167-174. Power appears in 1652.

39 Gotfredsen E, 'The Reception of Harvey's Doctrine in Denmark', *JHMAS*, 202-208.

[40] Ferrario E.V, 'William Harvey's Debate with Caspar Hofmann on the Circulation of the Blood', *JHMAS*, 15, (1960), 7-21.

[41] Lazare Riviere (Riverius) at Montpellier opposed Riolan and defended Harvey. Weil, 172.

[42] A transcript of the manuscript appears in Cole F.J, 'Henry Power on the Circulation of the Blood', *JHMAS*, 291-324.

[43] Cole F.J, 'Harvey's Animals', *JHMAS*, 106-113.

[44] All these bivalves have a well developed contracting heart.

[45] The absence of communication between the ventricles through the septum was essential in refuting Galen's account of the circulation.

[46] For a dog this seems excessive, but the point is: blood must circulate, otherwise a large quantity would have to be created and consumed.

Thomas Willis: 1621 - 1675

Willis created the word 'neurologie' which first appears, in Greek, in *Cerebri Anatome* in 1664, and, in English, in 1681.[1] The word 'neuro' comes from Greek for sinew or bowstring, which Willis recalled when dissecting the cranial, spinal, and autonomic nerves. His delineation of the peripheral and autonomic nervous systems was as great an advance as his discoveries in the brain and spinal cord.

Willis, born in 1621, lived most of his life in Oxford. The Civil War disrupted his classical studies and diverted him from theology to medicine: he graduated BM in 1646, endured the Protectorate under Oliver Cromwell, and

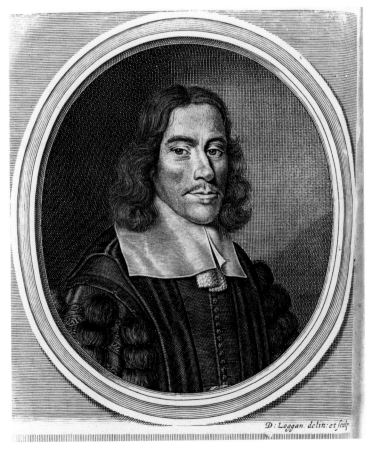

Figure 10.1 Engraving of Thomas Willis by David Loggan,
engraver to Oxford University from 1669. This appeared as the frontispiece facing
the title of *Pathologiae Cerebri*, 1667, J. Allestry, Oxford.

– a Royalist – was elevated in the Restoration of 1666, when King Charles II commanded his appointment to the Oxford Chair of Natural Philosophy. Willis taught medicine, but also anatomy, comparative anatomy, physiology, psychology, chemistry, and pharmacy.[2] From his lectures arose three textbooks in neuroscience: *Cerebri Anatome* on anatomy, *Pathologiae Cerebri* on pathology, and *De Anime Brutorum* on function. Interspersed in these were his own case reports and necropsies, with observations on anatomy, physiology, and pathology, and many descriptions of diseases and syndromes, some original.

Willis made many discoveries in neuroanatomy.[3] His were the first descriptions of the *nervus ophthalmicus Willisii*, the *nervus accessorium Willisii*, and the *Chordae Willisii* (trabeculae which traverse the meningeal sinuses). Anatomically, he distinguished the sympathetic nerves from the wandering (vagal) nerves, showing how both innervate the heart and arteries. His ligation of the vagi in a dog, producing cardiac irregularity, begins the physiological study of cardiac innervation. Willis was the first to describe and illustrate the brain from accurate observation, and his names – *e.g.* cerebral peduncles and medullary pyramids – persist. He described and illustrated the internal capsules and, in patients with long-standing hemiplegia, showed the unilateral capsular atrophy of cortico-spinal tract degeneration – the first description of tract degeneration. He was the first to describe the anterior commissure, the *stria terminalis*, the inferior olives, and the *claustrum*, and he made original studies of the spinal cord and its blood supply.[4]

Willis was as great a physician as an anatomist. In many diseases, his was the first clear description: in some, there is no previous account, as in *myasthenia gravis* (he hinted on its humoral cause), *akathisia* (restless legs syndrome), and *achalasia* of the *cardia*. In the last mentioned, he explained the disorder of physiology, and devised successful treatment with a probang, which he designed. *Paracusis Willisii* remains the diagnostic feature of stapes fixation. Eastern physicians had previously distinguished diabetes mellitus but Willis's description – in *Pharmaceutica Rationalis* – was the first in Europe, and his description of diabetic neuritis has no precedent.

I have selected eight necropsies from some twenty in Willis's textbooks – and these begin the specialty of neuropathology.[5] They consist of: 1. Congenital idiocy related to a small brain. 2. Stenosis of the carotid artery with enlargement of the ipsilateral vertebral artery – evidence that Willis appreciated the physiological importance of the circle named after him. 3. Frontal sinusitis progressing to pyogenic leptomeningitis and ventriculitis. 4. Congenital intracerebral haemorrhage. 5. Meningioma of the falx with obstruction of the veins and sinuses. 6. Venous thrombosis of the vein of Galen and straight sinus. 7. Subdural abscess arising from ear infection. 8. Sudden cerebral ischaemia from cardiac arrest.

Willis died in London in 1675, and is buried in Westminster Abbey. Self taught, he was a pioneer in neurology and founder of several of the neurosciences.

REFERENCES

[1] Willis, T. *Cerebri Anatome cui accessit Nervorum descriptio et usus*, typis Ja. Flesher, impensis Jo. Martyn & Ja. Allestry *Londini*: 1664. Translated into English by Pordage, S. London: T. Dring, C. Harper, J. Leigh, and S. Martyn, 1681.

[2] John Locke attended Willis's lectures and his notes have been translated, edited, and published in: Dewhurst, K. *Thomas Willis's Oxford Lectures*. Oxford: Sandford Publications, Oxford, 1980.

[3] Meyer, A. *Historical Aspects of Cerebral Anatomy*. London: Oxford University Press, 1971.

[4] Hughes, J.T. (1982) Spinal cord arteries described by Willis. Chapter 20 in: *Historical aspects of the Neurosciences*, edited by F.C. Rose and W.F. Bynum. New York: Raven Press, 1982.

[5] Hughes, J.T, 'Thomas Willis: the first Oxford Neuropathologist'. In: *Neuroscience Across the Centuries*, edited by F.C. Rose. London: Smith-Gordon, 1989.

Thomas Willis: the First Oxford Neuropathologist.

The story of Thomas Willis (Figure 11.1) begins with his birth in Great Bedwyn, (Figure 11.2) in Wiltshire in 1621 (Symonds and Feindel, 1969),[1] and ends in London where he died in 1675, being buried in Westminster Abbey (Feindel, 1962).[2] It was, however, in Oxford that he carried out most of his important work and, of the 54 years of his life, about 30 were spent in Oxford. He lived for most of his childhood at North Hinksey near Oxford, and went to the private school of Edward Sylvester in High street, Oxford, and subsequently, at the age of 15 years, to the college of Christ Church of the University of Oxford. During his adult life in Oxford, he lived with his wife and children in a house, still standing, in Merton street, opposite Merton College, and called Beam Hall. In 1666 he moved to a lucrative medical practice in London, but most of his famous writings were based

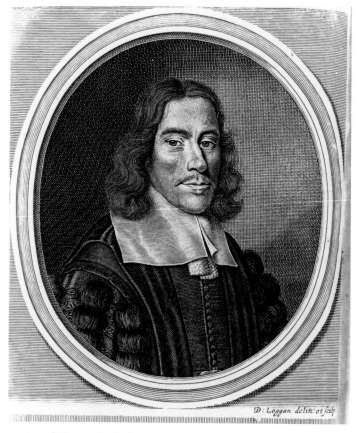

D: Loggan delin: et sculp

Figure 11.1 Engraving of Thomas Willis by David Loggan, engraver to Oxford University from 1669. This appeared as the frontispiece facing the title of *Pathologiae Cerebri*, 1667, J. Allestry, Oxford.

on his extensive medical experience in Oxford and also on his anatomical studies and animal experiments, mostly carried out whilst he occupied the chair of Natural Philosophy of the University of Oxford. For short biographies of Willis, the introductory chapter of the modern edition of *Cerebri Anatome* by Feindel (Willis, 1965),[3] the account, in the Dictionary of Scientific Biography, by Frank (1976),[4] and the biographical notes preceding Willis' lectures published by the late Kenneth Dewhurst (Dewhurst, 1980)[5] are recommended. There is a full biography by Isler (1965, 1968).[6] I have made extensive use of the important bibliography compiled by Wing (1962).[7]

The modern reputation of Thomas Willis is mainly that of an anatomist with a specialised interest in neuroanatomy, then little understood (Meyer, 1966).[8] However, his contributions to comparative anatomy (Cole, 1944),[9] to physiology (Meyer and Hierons, 1965;[10] Brazier, 1984),[11] and to experimental pathology were of equal importance. As a physician, his reputation suffered from the judgement of a few of his contemporaries, some envious of his successful medical practice in London. His reputation was also denigrated by the comments of his contemporary, Anthony Wood, who seems to have nurtured an intense personal dislike of Willis. My judgement is that, as a physician, he ranks amongst the first in the seventeenth century. Evidence of this ranking is that he is credited with at least six disease states, in which he provided, for those times, the first clear account of the disease, with which he was familiar from his own clinical observation. One reason for his modest posthumous fame, is that, whilst his original clinical observations were numerous, they did not include any single discovery of the magnitude of those of Harvey and some other contemporaries.

Many of his medical discoveries arose from his habit of clinico-pathological correlation. He made detailed notes, in Latin, of the clinical features of his cases. If the outcome was fatal, he or his assistants frequently performed an autopsy, the findings of which he recorded in detail. He had a particular interest in diseases of the nervous system, being one of the first specialists in this field and, indeed, creating the name neurology for the subject. It follows that many of his autopsy reports are the first neuropathological accounts of many diseases of the brain. Even when an earlier description of a neurological disease exists, that of Willis is often more detailed, and more precise, especially in referring to the anatomical structures that were found to be pathologically abnormal. Here his interest and knowledge of anatomy contributed greatly to the significance of his observations. Finally, in the cases with necropsy described by Willis, there is usually an excellent clinical account, not always present in earlier recorded case reports, and this account is the more valuable because it often derives from his own case notes, and gives his own observations and clinical opinion on the case. My title names Willis as the first Oxford neuropathologist, but he has claims to be one of the first neuropathologists in the world.

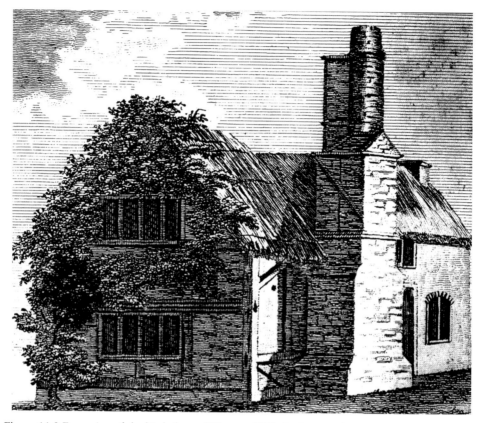

Figure 11.2 Engraving of the birthplace of Thomas Willis in Great Bedwyn, Wiltshire, reproduced from the Gentleman's Magazine of 1798. Courtesy of the Bodleian Library, Oxford.

The published works of Thomas Willis

The works of Thomas Willis were published in seven separate books all in Latin, except for the last, which was published in English, in 1691, after the author's death. These seven works are so important that I shall list them chronologically with some comments derived from the researches of H. J. R.Wing (Wing, 1962).[7]

1. *Diatribae duae medico-philosophicae.* 1659. This, the first of Willis' major works, was published first in London in an octavo edition. There were many subsequent editions from London, The Hague, and Amsterdam. The work consists of two tracts, one on Fermentation, the other on Fevers, to which is added a dissertation on Urine.

2. *Cerebri Anatome.* 1664. The '*Cerebri Anatome cui accessit Nervorum descriptio et usus*' (Figure 11.3) was first published in London in a quarto edition. There were many subsequent London editions and then several from Amsterdam. At the time of its first appearance, it was recognised as an important new anatomical work, which made Willis famous throughout Europe in the field of

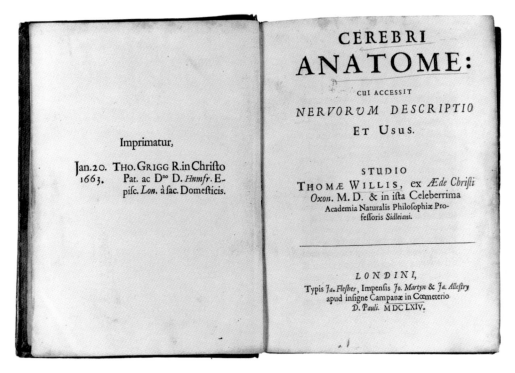

Figure 11.3 Title page of *Cerebri Anatome*. Figs 11.2-11.6 are photographs taken by Mr M.R. Dudley of copies in the library of Christ Church, Oxford.

medical and biological research. In my opinion, it is the best and most important work of Willis. Critics of Willis, notably his contemporary Anthony Wood, stated that others and in particular Richard Lower, the pupil of Willis, and also Christopher Wren, helped in the work and deserve most of the credit. This criticism has been adequately refuted, and for discussion on this point, the 1955 Harveian Oration of Sir Charles Symonds (Symonds,1955)[12] should be consulted.

3. *Pathologiae cerebri*. 1667. The '*Pathologiae cerebri et nervosi generis specimen*' (Figure 11.4) was the succeeding work promised by Willis in the *Cerebri anatome* and was first published in a quarto edition at Oxford in 1667. Subsequent editions were printed in London and Amsterdam. This also was a very important work, well received by european doctors and scientists, and further enhancing the reputation of Willis. The work contains several crucial case reports describing diverse diseases some with the first ever recorded clear description. The neuropathological content of this work and of the *Cerebri Anatome* will be described in detail later.

4. *Affectionum quae dicuntur hystericae et hypochondriacae*. 1670. This work was first published in a quarto edition in London in 1670. Subsequently, further editions appeared from Leyden and London. The work is in three parts dealing in turn with hysteria, blood, and muscular action.

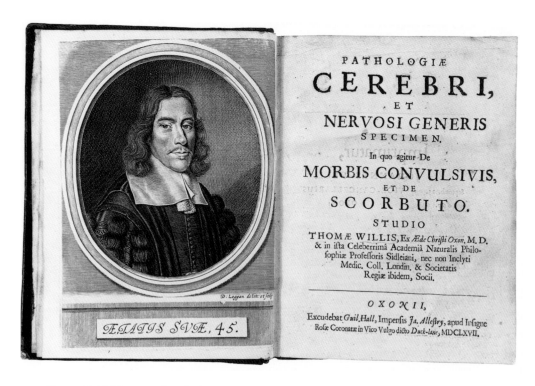

Figure 11.4 Title page of *Pathologiae Cerebri*. The engraving of Thomas Willis is by Loggan.

5. *De anima brutorum quae hominis vitalis ac sensitiva est* .1672. The '*De anima brutorum*' (Figure 11.5) was first published in a quarto edition in Oxford in 1672 and again in the same year in an octavo edition in London and Amsterdam. There were many subsequent editions providing evidence of the contemporary reputation of the work. This book is one of the great works of medical science and was considered by Willis his most important publication. It was written in solitude after the tragic death of his wife, and abounds with important clinical observations, some with the first description of a disease state. The neuropathological content of this important work will be described in detail below.

6. *Pharmaceutice rationalis*. 1674-1675. This work is in two parts, the first, published at Oxford in 1674, and the second part, usually bound separately, published, also at Oxford, posthumously in 1675. The imprimatur of the second part is dated November 12th, 1675, the day after the death of Willis. Amongst a miscellany of observations and speculations, there are historically important statements on pharmacological remedies, alimentary function, diabetes, tobacco and coffee taking, respiratory disease, blood letting, and various skin conditions.

7. *A plain and easie method of preserving those that are well from the plague*. 1691. This work first appeared as an octavo edition in London in 1691, sixteen

years after the death of Willis. It was a compilation edited from the manuscripts of Willis and contains a number of prescriptions. It is the only major work of Willis to be published in English.

Of the seven books listed above, three, the *Cerebri anatome*, the *Pathologiae cerebri*, and the *De anima brutorum* are of the greatest importance in the development of understanding of anatomy, physiology and human diseases. They form an interesting triology, planned in this form by Willis, of which the first dealt with the anatomy of the brain, the second with the pathology of the brain, whilst the last is concerned with the soul or psyche.

The Case Reports

Reading again these three great works for their content of neuropathology, I have found some 20 case reports with a necropsy reported in sufficient detail to be worthy of study. From these I have chosen eight for description and discussion here. I shall first give the original Latin text with the correction of obvious errors, then my English translation, and finally a comment on the case. I am indebted to an Oxford colleague, Mr. J.H.C.Leach of Pembroke College, for checking my translations.

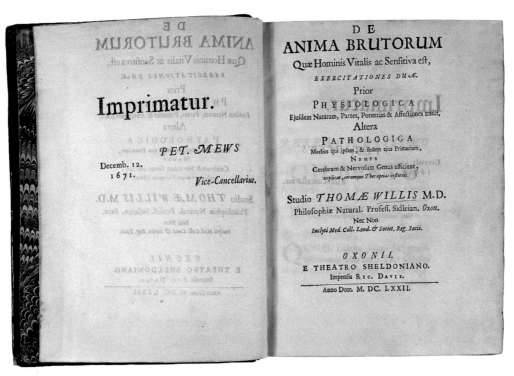

Figure 11.5 Title page of *De Anima Brutorum*.

Case 1. (Figure 11.6a) (From fig 1111 of the *Cerebri anatome*. and the legend)

Effigies Cerebri humani, quod cujusdam Adolescentis, ab ipsa nativitate Fatui, &
ex eorum numero qui vulgo Lemurum subdititii perhibentur, fuerat; Cujus Cerebri
moles, cum tenuior ac solito minor fuit, limbus ejus ulterius elevari & reflecti
potuit, ut interiora quaevis penitus conspicerentur.

(Figure 11.6b) The drawing of a human brain of a certain youth that was foolish
from his birth, and of the sort which are commonly termed changelings. The
limbus could be lifted up and turned back to permit a good view of the interior.

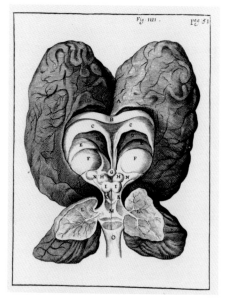

Figure 11.6a Fig 1111 on page 51 of *Cerebri Anatome*, illustrating our case 1.

Figura Quarta.

Effigies Cerebri humani, quod cujufdam A-
dolefcentis, ab ipfa nativitate Fatui, & ex
eorum numero qui vulgò Lemurum fub-
dititii perhibentur, fuerat; Cujus Cerebri moles, cùm tenuior ac folito minor fuit, limbus ejus ulteriùs elevari & reflecti
potuit, ut interiora quævis penitiùs confpi-
cerentur.

Figure 11.6b Latin text referring to our case 1.

This case report describes congenital idiocy with a small brain.

Case 2. (Figure 11.7) (From the *Cerebri anatome.* Pages 95 and 96) *Non ita pridem cujusdam defuncti cadaver dissecuimus, quem schirrus intra mesenterium ingens, ac demum ulcerosus, extinxerat: in eo, dum cranio aperto, quae ad* ἐγκέφαλον *pertinebant lustravimus, carotidem dextram intra cranium emergentem, plane osseam, seu potius lapideam (cavitate ejus fere in totum occlusa) invenimus; adeo ut sanguinis influxu hac via denegato, mirum videatur quare aeger non prius interiisset Apoplecticus: quod equidem in tantum abfuit, ut mentis suae, & functionis animalis libero exercitio usque ad extremum vitae momentum potiretur. Enimvero contra illud Apoplexiae periculum, natura remedium satis idoneum substituerat; nimirum ex eodem latere quo carotis defecerat, Arteria vertebralis, Tubuli mole aucta, pari sua alterius lateris triplo*

Non ità pridem cujufdam defuncti cadaver diffecuimus, quem *fchirrus* intra mefenterium ingens, ac demum ulcerofus, extinxerat : in eo, dum cranio aperto, quæ ad ἐγκέφαλον pertinebant luftravimus, *carotidem dextram* intra cranium emergentem, planè *offeam,* feu potiùs *lapideam* (cavitate ejus ferè in totum occlufâ) invenimus ; adeò ut fanguinis influxu hâc viâ denegato, mirum videatur quare æger non priùs interiiffet Apoplecticus: quod equidem in tantum abfuit, ut mentis *fuæ,* & functionis animalis libero exercitio ufque ad extremum vitæ momentum potiretur. Enimvero contra illud Apoplexiæ periculum, natura remedium fatìs idoneum fubftituerat ; nimirum ex eodem latere quo *carotis defecerat, Arteria vertebralis,* Tubuli mole auctâ, *pari fuâ* alterius lateris *triplo major evaferat:* Quippe fanguis *Carotide* exclufus, vertebralis folito vectigali fefe infuper addens, & duplicato fluvio in eundem alveum confluens, arteriæ iftius canalem ità fupra modum

Figure 11.7 Latin text of case 2, complete save the last word.

major evaserat: Quippe sanguis Carotide exclusus, vertebralis solito vectigali sese insuper addens, & duplicato fluvio in eundem alveum confluens, arteriae istius canalem ita supra modum dilataverat.

It is not long since we dissected the cadaver of a certain man, who died of a large scirhous tumour of the mesentery, which became ulcerated. When his skull was opened we noted amongst the usual intracranial findings, the right carotid artery, in its intracranial part, bony or even stony hard, its lumen being being almost totally occluded; so that the influx of blood being denied by this route, it seemed remarkable that this person had not died previously of an apoplexy: which indeed he was so far from, that he enjoyed to the last moments of his life, the free exercise of his mental and bodily functions. For indeed, nature had provided a sufficient remedy against the risk of apoplexy in the vertebral artery of the same side in which the carotid was wanting, since the size of this vessel was enlarged, becoming thrice that of the contralateral vessel: the reason being that because the blood was excluded from the carotid, the required flow added to the perfusion of the vertebral, and flowing in that lumen in twice the amount had enlarged that vessel beyond the normal.

This important account includes the essential clinical record that the patient had normal mental and physical functions before his death from an abdominal tumour. The detailed description of the stenosed carotid artery, and the consequent enlargement of the ipsilateral vertebral artery is part of the evidence that Willis appreciated, not only the anatomy of the arterial circle named after him, but its physiological importance.

Case 3. (From the *Cerebri anatome*. Pages 151 and 152)

Non ita pridem Virgo, in hac urbe degens, cephalea immani diu assligebatur, atque inter medios cruciatus, multum seri flavl & tenuis quotidie naribus essluebat: novissima hyeme haec excretio aliquandiu substitit, & tunc demum aegrotans, & capitate deterius habente, in convulsiones atroces cum stupore incidebat; atque intra triduum apoplectica interibat. Capite aperto, latex ejusmodi flavus Cerebri anfractus profundiores, ejusque cavitatem interiorem seu ventriculos, inundabat.

A virgin living in this city, was afflicted a long time with a most cruel headache, and in the midst of her pain much thin yellowish secretions flowed daily from her nostrils: last winter this excretion ceased for a while, and then becoming sick in the head, she developed violent convulsions, with accompaning stupor, and within three days died in apoplexy. On opening the skull, a yellowish exudate covered the sulci of the brain, and also filled the interior cavities called ventricles.

This case, of a type still common in Oxford, where the damp atmosphere of the Thames valley predisposes to upper respiratory infections, has the clinical course and pathological findings of frontal sinusitis progressing to a pyogenic leptomeningitis and ventriculitis.

Case 4. (From *Pathologiae cerebri*. Pages 49 and 50)

In this chapter Willis is discussing convulsions in infants soon after birth.

Olim in hac urbe cujusdam mulieris nati plures ex hoc morbo interierunt; tandem Faetus quarti intra mensem, uti priores, interempti, caput dissecuimus, nulla hic serosa colluvies ventriculos inundabat, sed cerebri tantum, ejusque appendicic substantia erat justo humidior, & laxior: quod potissimum observatu dignum erat, in cavitate quae cerebello subjicitur, supra medullae oblongatae caudicem, sanguinis grumosi, & velut concreti copiam insignem reperiebamus: at vero incertum est utrum materies istaec ibidem ab initio deposita spasmos primario intulerat; an potius sanguis iste a partium circumeirea consitarum contractione expressus, & extravasatus, convulsionum effectus, & productum, ac minime istarum fuerit; Nam & in Apoplecticis ejusmodi Phaenomenon passim occurrit; quod tamen morbi essectum potius quam causam esse posthaec ostendemus.

Sometime past in this city, more children of a certain woman died of this disease, at length, the fourth, as the others died within a month. We dissected the head of this fourth offspring, and found no serous collection or excess watery fluid overflowing from the ventricles, but only that the substance of the brain was moister and more diffluent than normal. What was most significant was that, in the ventricular cavity, within the cerebrum, lying on the floor, was a remarkable heap of clotted, and as it were, concreted blood. In truth it is uncertain, whether this matter, deposited there from the begining, had primarily caused the convulsions; or rather, whether, this blood being extravasated, and expressed, from the structures around, was not the effeet, and product of the convulsions, rather than the cause of them; for also in apoplectical people this kind of phenomenon ordinarily happens, which yet we shall afterwards shew, to be rather the effect, than the cause of the disease.

This is a case of congenital intracerebral haemorrhage, a condition still with unexplained features. Note how Willis excludes a meningitis (no serous collection) and hydrocephalus ('no' excess watery fluid) with which he was evidently familiar. He notes the similar pathology found in intracerebral haemorrhage in adults and his uncertainty whether the haemorrhage is the primary event.

Case 5. (From *De Anima Brutorum*. Pages 296 - 297)

Mulier quinquagenaria postguam per sex circiter menses gravissimo capitis dolore, sub sutura sagattali eam perpetuotere molestante, nullique medicamentis, aut methodo cedente, laborasset, tandem in lethargum cum membrorum resolutione partiali incidit, a quibus tamen' per remedia tempestive adhibita brevi recuperata in cephalgiam uti prius atrocem expergiscebatur, porro deinde intra duas, vel tres septimanas, in assectionem soporosam relapsa evita discessit. Cranio aperto e latere sinus tertii, tumor scirrhosus tres digitos latus membranis accreverat, cujus interventu & dura meninx aliquanto spatio piae accreverat, & vasa sanguifera, quae illic in sinus cavitatem dehiscere debuerunt, constipabantur.

A woman of about fifty years of age, after she had borne for about six months, a most grievous pain in the head, under the sagittal suture (or the seam that goes through the length of the skull, dividing it into two parts), troubling her almost continually, yielding to no medicines or regime of treatment, finally fell into a lethargy, with a partial alleviation of her symptoms; from which being aroused by remedies, she awoke with the headache, as distressing as before. Within two or three weeks later, relapsing again into stupor, she departed this life. Her skull being opened, there was growing from the side of the sagittal sinus, a scirrhous tumor three fingers broad, which united for a small area the dura mater to the pia mater, and the venous tributaries, which should open here into the sinus, were occluded.

This case, of a meningioma of the falx, is described, although with an economy of words, with such clarity that the diagnosis is certain. Willis was also aware of the obstruction to the venous drainage and the sinuses of these tumours and the clinical effect of this is dealt with in the succeeding passages.

Case 6. (From De Anima Brutorum, pages 301 and 302)

Olim juvenis Academicus cum per duas septimas de gravissimo capitis dolore ipsum incessanter affligente conquestus, erat tandem febre aucta, mox vigiliae, motus convulsivi, ac confabulatio delira succedebant; quo tempore medicus accersitus, phlebotomia, enematis, emplastris, revulsivis, vesicatoriis, item remediis internis, quae fluxionem sanguinis, ac humorunia capite devocent, sedulo adhibitis, nihil proficere potuit, quin mors brevi successerit. Calvaria aperta, vasa meningas obducentia erant sanguine repleta, & plurimum distenta, quasi cruoris massa illuc tota confluxerat, ita ut sinibus dissectis, & apertis, cruor assatim erumpens, ad plures uncias, supra lib.fs. pondus essluxerit: porro ipsae membrane, tumore phlegmonide per totum assectae, discolores apparebant.

Some time ago, a young university man, after complaining for two weeks of severe pain in the head, constantly present, developed a fever, from which he awoke with convulsions and incoherent speech. By now a physician had been summoned who administered bleeding, enemas, plasters, emetics, blistering, and internal remedies designed to draw blood from the head. These remedies, although carefully administered, were of no value and death followed. His skull being opened, the vessels leading to the meninges were filled with blood, and very much distended, as if the whole content of blood had gathered there, so that , the venous sinuses, being opened by dissection, the blood gushed out and flowed to a weight of several ounces greater than half a pint. Also, the leptomeninges themselves were abnormal throughout with an inflammatory discoloured swelling.

This case of acute fever progressing to convulsions and death from cerebral compression seems due to venous infarction, possibly caused by an obstruction of the vein of Galen or the straight sinus. A septic thrombosis is a likely cause of the obstruction.

Case 7. (From De anima Brutorum, page 302)

Memini alium Academicum, qui post diuturnam hemicraniam, sub sutura temporali, per tres septimanas eum perpetuo, & gravissime assligentem, in Apoplexiam brevi funestam incidit. Capite aperto phlegmon juxta locum dolentem in menigibus accreveret, a qua demum suppurata, & disrupta, sanies in cerebrum deciden, substantiam ejus livore & putedine assecerat.

I remember another academic, who after a prolonged one sided headache, under the temporal suture, and constantly present for three weeks, rapidly developed a fatal apoplexy. When the cranium was opened, an inflammatory swelling had arisen in the meninges, near the position of the head pain, and from the bursting of this suppuration, the underlying brain had been discoloured by the putrefaction.

This is another case of cerebral inflammation and possibly a subdural abcess, which, from its position, may have been related to ear infection.

Case 8. (From De Anima Brutorum, pages (389-391)

Senex Theologus, vir probus, & pius, corpore obeso, nec non collo breviori, & toroso praeditus, diu invaletudinarius, & vitam sedentariam agens, cacochmiam valde scorbuticam contraxerat: respiratione dissicili, & anhelosa, & capitis gravitate, & torpore insolito assectus, vix quicquam praeterea laboris, aut exercitii praestare poterat, quam quod quotidie e cubiculo ad Sacellum, & Refectorium iret, & rediret. Quodam mane Capellam paulo ante preces ingressus, dum genibus provolvitur, derepente perculsus, & mox , & insensilis factus, in humum concidit, illico vero sublatus, & vestibus exutus, lecto concalfacto imponitur. Ipse, alique medici mox accersiti, ac ocyssime adventantes reperimus eum, non modo absq, sensu, pulsu, & respiratione sed toto corpore frigentem, & plane rigidum, nec ullis remediis, aut administrationum modis aliquandiu licet diligentissime adhibitis, ad vitam aut incalescentiam revocari potuit: unde suspicati sumus a primo ictu, cordis pulsum penitus ihibitum fuisse, flammaq; ejus extincta, sanguinis statim omnem motum suppressum fuisse. Postridie Cadaver exanime satis, & obriguisse visum, aperuimus, nihil dubitantes, quin affectus itasubito lethalis, vestigia satis clara, intra relicta, in conspectum prodierint. Verum illic, aut in alia quavis parte, morbi licet atrocissimi, ne vel umbra quaedam supererat.

An ancient divine, an honest and godly man, but blessed with an obese frame, with a short brawny neck, being long unhealthy, and living a sedentary life, developed a serious scorbutic syndrome, characterised by laboured breathing, heaviness of the head, and a feeling of numbness, was scarcely able to undertake any labour or exercise, more than his daily attendance at chapel and hall from his chamber. One morning he came to the chapel a little before prayers had commenced, and, whilst he was on his knees, he was suddenly struck by an immediate loss of speech and conciousness, and fell to the ground. He was carried thence, his clothes were removed, and he was placed into a warm bed. I and other physicians, being sent for, and coming as soon as possible, found him not only without pulse, sense and breathing, but the body cold and quite stiff, nor could he be recalled to life by any remedies or procedures, in spite of their prolonged administration. We suspected that the pulse of the heart was wholly arrested at the onset of his stroke, and because its flame was extinguished, presently all motion of the circulation ceased. The next day, seeing the body dead and stiff, we opened it, not doubting but that the sudden fatal illness would show clear evidence of its nature within the head. But there, or indeed elsewhere, was no trace of the cause of this malign disease.

Then follows a lengthy description of the brain and its vessels, meninges and ventricles, giving evidence of the thorough intracranial inspection practised by Willis. He then describes his general necropsy findings begining 'lest the cause should lie hid somewhere without the head' finding acute pulmonary oedema but little else. He speculates, concluding with a diagnosis of cardiac arrest ' the motion of the heart failing, like the prime wheel of a clock or watch, immediately all other functions, their impulses being taken away, wholly ceased.'

This necropsy account, my own favorite, shows the accurate observation of Willis, truly describing his findings despite the puzzling absence of gross intracranial pathology. The problem remains today for the pathologist who expecting to find cerebral haemorrhage or infarction in a case of stroke eventually concludes that sudden cerebral ischaemia from a cardiac arrest is the primary pathological event (Hughes, 1985).[13]

The Neuropathological Necropsy

The development of the necropsy in Europe as an aid to medical enlightment is complex, since, for many centuries, cadavers were opened and the organs inspected from several motives. In this report, we are less concerned with the development of the teaching of anatomy by dissection, although naturally many pathological features were discovered in this way. The great Italian painters of the Renaissance were seeking anatomical knowledge and sometimes attended dissections on persons dying in the hospitals of Florence, Milan and Rome, and incidentally, illustrating with great artistic skill some abnormal pathological appearance. In this survey we are more concerned with the development of the autopsy as a tool of enquiry in medical science.

By the thirteenth century, physicians in Italy were conducting autopsies in cases of suspicious death, usually when poisoning was suspected. One of the earliest autopsies for this reason in Italy was that conducted by Guglielmo da Varignana at Bologna in 1302, and in France probably the first judicial autopsy was performed by Ambrose Paré in 1562. By the mid seventeenth century, necropsies to ascertain the cause of death were probably common throughout Europe. There is space here to mention only a few early morbid anatomists comparable to Willis.

William Harvey (1578-1657), who was both Warden of Merton College, Oxford, and physician to the King during the Civil War, performed many autopsies, and probably influenced Willis, and many other doctors then in Oxford towards this method of medical research, whilst Francis Glisson (1597-1677) was similarly active in Cambridge. Elsewhere in europe the necropsy flourished in the new Dutch republic, where in Amsterdam, Nicholas Tulp (1593-1674) made important observations on cancers, and many other disease states. Franciscus de la Boe Sylvius (1614-1672), described the pathology of tuberculosis, having performed innumerable autopsies at Leyden, where was to be found, for nine years, Thomas Bartholin (1616-1680), before he returned to his native Copenhagen. Rivalling Willis in a special interest in the brain was Johann Jakob Wepfer of Shaffhausen (1620 – 1695), who described the pathological appearances of cerebral haemorrhage. In Italy, there was Marcello Malpighi (1628-1694) in Pisa pursuing the new subject of histology as an extension of macroscopic pathology, and when in 1694, he died of apoplexy, his own autopsy was performed by his pupil Giogio Baglivi (1669-1707).

It is interesting to compare these accounts with those of Willis, whose descriptions were mainly earlier in that century. However, this account does not claim that the 8 necropsies of Willis, detailed here, all made new pathological observations, but rather that they form a considerable body of evidence of the extent of Willis's knowledge of neuropathology in the 17th century.

I close this brief account of the flourishing of necropsies in the 17th century, with mention of Theophile Bonet (1620-1689), who, born in Geneva, and qualifying in Bologna, became physician to the Duc de Longueville, and occupied many years of leisurely practice in compiling an account of notable necropsies from Hippocrates to his own time, although naturally those of the 16th and 17th centuries predominated. This immense publication called the 'Sepulchretum',[14] is a thesaurus of necropsies, amongst them many performed by Willis, the first Oxford Neuropathologist.

ACKNOWLEDGEMENTS

I am grateful to Mr H.J.R. Wing, librarian at Christ Church, Oxford, for making available to me editions of Willis's works, and allowing me to quote from his bibliography[7], to Mr J.T. Leach, of Pembroke College, Oxford, for checking my Latin translations, and to Mr M.R. Dudley of the Ashmolean Museum, Oxford for his expert photography. I thank Dr A.H.T. Robb-Smith for many discussions on Willis and his work.

REFERENCES

[1] Symonds, C. and Feindel,W. 'Birthplace of Thomas Willis', *British Medical Journal, 2* (1969), 648-649.

[2] Feindel, W. 'Restoration of the Memorial to Dr. Thomas Willis' (1621-1675) in Westminster Abbey, *British Medical Journal, 1* (1962), 552.

[3] Willis, T. The Anatomy of the Brain and Nerves, Tercentenary edition, edited by William Feindel. Montreal: McGill University Press, 1965.

[4] Frank, R.G. Jr., 'Thomas Willis'. In, *Dictionary of Scientific Biography' XIV.* New York: Charles Scribner's Sons, 1970-1976, 404-409.

[5] Dewhurst, K. *Thomas Willis's Oxford Lectures.* Oxford: Sandford Publications, 1980.

[6] Isler, H-R. *Thomas Willis 1621-1675, Doctor and Scientist.* New York: Hafner, 1968. Translated by the author with additions from the original 1965 German edition, Band 29 of Grosse Naturforcher, published by Wissenschaftliche Verlagsgesellschaft m.b.H., Stuttgart: 1965.

[7] Wing, H.J.R. A bibliography of Dr. Thomas Willis 1975). Thesis, University of London Diploma in Librarianship, 1962.

[8] Meyer, A. 'Karl Friedrich Burdach on Thomas Willis', *Journal of Neurological Science,* 3, (1971), 109-116.

[9] Cole, F.J. *A history of comparative anatomy from Aristotle to the eighteenth century.* London: 1944.

[10] Meyer, A. and Hierons, R. 'On Thomas Willis's concepts of neurophysiology', *Medical History,* 9, (1965), 1-15.

[11] Brazier, M.A.B. *A history of neurophysiology in the 17th and 18th centuries.* New York, Raven Press, 63-66, 1984.

[12] Symonds, G. 'The Circle of Willis', *British Medical Journal,* 1 (1955), 119-124.

[13] Hughes, J.T., Necropsies on patients after stroke. *British Medical Journal, 291,* (1985), 843.

[14] Bonet, T. (1679). *Sepulchretum, sive anatomia practica ex cadaveribus morbo denati.* Genevae: L. Chouet.

Spinal Cord Arteries Described by Willis

Thomas Willis is well known for his descriptions of the anatomy of the brain based on dissections and detailed examinations of most of the components of the brain with an important description of the cranial and spinal nerves. What is less recognized is that his publications include the first accurate descriptions of the vascular supply of the spinal cord. The present chapter singles out this part of his work from the better known account of the anatomy of the brain in his book *Cerebri Anatome: cui accessit Nervorum Descriptio et Usus*, published in 1664.

Thomas Willis and his Colleagues

During his active research period in Oxford, Willis had as associates or pupils a remarkable group of scientific workers. Among these were Robert Hooke, John Locke, Edmund King, William Petty, Richard Lower, Thomas Millington, and Christopher Wren. In that part of Willis' work that concerns the anatomy of the blood vessels of the spinal cord, Richard Lower took a prominent part, and Thomas Millington and Christopher Wren were involved to a lesser degree.

Thomas Willis was born in 1621 in Great Bedwyn in Wiltshire but moved as a boy to North Hinksey near Oxford. He came as a pupil to Christchurch, Oxford, in 1636, graduated B.A. in 1639 and M.A. in 1642. After the disturbances of the civil war, he returned to Oxford, where he set up medical practice and was appointed Sedleian Professor of Natural Philosophy in 1660. His researches on neurological anatomy date from this period, and his famous book *Cerebri Anatome* was published in 1664. He moved to London in 1667 where he died in 1675 of pneumonia.

Richard Lower was born in 1631 and, like Willis, was educated at Christchurch, Oxford, proceeding to M.A. in 1655 and M.D. in 1665. It is clear from Willis' writings and also from letters of Richard Lower that a great part of the anatomical dissection and some of the drawings in *Cerebri Anatome* were done by Lower. Willis himself in the preface to his book gives fulsome acknowledgment:

> And here I made use of the Labours of the most Learned Physician and highly skilled Anatomist, Dr. Richard Lower, for my help and Companion; the edge of whose Knife and Wit I willingly acknowledge to have been a help to me for the better searching out both the frame and offices of before hidden Bodies.

Sir Christopher Wren (1632-1723), originally a pupil of Willis, made many of the drawings in Willis' book. He probably did not draw those that illustrated the vascular supply of the spinal cord, which probably were drawn by Lower. At the time of this collaboration, Wren was Savilian Professor of Astronomy at Oxford and, from mathematics, astronomy, and science, he was now turning to architecture, being busy with the designs of the new Sheldonian Theatre. One further contribution of Wren should be noted. Wren devised various techniques for carrying out intravenous injections in animals, and these methods were used in the first successful blood transfusion in man by Richard Lower and Edmund King. Injections of india ink and other fluids were used with considerable advantage by both Willis and Lower to show up the blood vessels to the brain and spinal cord. Wren contributed by advice and assistance in these injection studies.

Thomas Millington (1628-1704) graduated at Trinity College, Cambridge, and moved to Oxford in 1657 when he took his M.D. He was elected a Fellow of All Souls in 1659. In the preface to his book, Willis describes the contribution of Millington and Wren in terms that suggest that their contribution was equal. He said

> it becomes me not to hide how much besides I did receive from these most famous Men, Dr. Thomas Millington, Doctor in Physick and Dr. Chr Wren, Doctor of Laws and Savill Professor of Astronomy; both which were wont frequently to be present at our Dissections and to confer and reason about the uses of the Parts. Besides the former most Learned Man, to whom I from day to day proposed privately my Conjectures and Observations, often confirmed me by his Suffrage, being uncertain in my mind, and not trusting to my own opinion. But the other most renowned Man, Dr. Wren, was pleased out of his singular humanity, wherewith he abounds, to delineate with his own most skillful hands many Figures of the Brain and Skull, whereby the work might be more exact".

To summarize the distribution of work, Willis appears to have been the originator and driving force behind the anatomical work, Richard Lower was the skillful prosector, preparing and injecting specimens and possibly drawing some of them, and Christopher Wren made a major contribution by his technique of injecting, and also in the drawings, some of which have a distinctive style attributed to him. Millington was an anatomist of profound knowledge and was of considerable help in discussion on the structure and function of the brain.

The Anatomical Work

The work of anatomical dissection was based on necropsies of patients, and these frequently had been in the practice of the group of doctors concerned. In some accounts, symptoms and signs of a terminal illness are given, and in one famous example, the necropsy revealed a cerebral hemorrhage. Doubtless these necropsies were used as opportunities for anatomical dissection. Preservation of the tissue was probably obtained by the use of spirits of wine, which was pioneered by Robert Boyle in Oxford. Willis and Lower probably injected the preservative into the vessels as well as using it for immersion, a considerable advance in preserving the brain, which consequently was spared the distortion evident in earlier work. The examination of the spinal arteries was far from easy.

Willis writes:

> But by what means these Vessels proceed on both sides from the Trunk of the Vertebral artery, and also the blood-carrying Veins, which are destinated to the whole spinal Marrow. and the inferior portion of its arterious passages, doth not so plainly appear; because the boney Cloisters of the Vertebra are not broken through without much labour. especially in grown up living Creatures: and in that work the beginnings and branchings out of very many Vessels are want to be blotted out.

Willis resorted, as many have since, to fetal material:

> But that we might more accurately search in these hid things, we made the Dissections of several Embryons, in which we are able to dissect the Vertebrae as yet soft, and to take out of them the Marrow whole, and look more narrowly into all the recesses of the bones.

Willis and Lower indicate clearly the success of their injection experiments by this passage:

> "...further, that all the tracts and branchings out of them might be the better perceived in all the Vessels, we did cast in divers coloured Liquors. And we had our desired wish: for presently we found with much admiration, that those kind of vessels, viz. arteries, Bosoms, and veins which respect the head, belong also the spinal manrow with no less a noted disposition of provision". Willis is clear that the vertebral arteries not only supply the hinder part of the brain but also the upper part of the spinal cord. "But the Vertebral Artery pays to the superior part of the Spine as great Tributes of Blood as to the Head itself." Willis also understood that while the vertebral arteries supplied the upper part of the spinal cord, the supply below came directly from the aorta. The following passage is crucial: "The Arteries which carry the Blood toward the Spine, are disposed after one manner above the Heart, and after another below it. As to the first, whereas the Trunk of the Aorta being there cleft presently to many branches departs from the Region of the Spine, theretore the Vertebral Artery is produced on both sides from its axillary branches, which ascending straight into the hinder part of the Head sends forth a branch into the meeting together of every

Vertebra. But below the Heart, forasmuch as the Aorta, in its whole descent, lyeth on the Spine, two arteries are received into the Spine from its bottom nigh its Internodia or spaces between the knots of the Vertebrae; so that if the trunk of the Aorta be cut open long-ways, there will appear a series of double holes through its whole tract.

The Anatomical Illustrations

The pictures of the spinal cord vascular supply appear in tables 12 and 13. Table 12 Figure 12.1 is an anterior aspect of the spinal cord seen after the dura has been

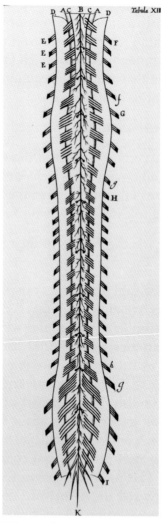

Figure 12.1 Table XII from Willis *Cerebri Anatome* (1664). The figure shows the anterior aspect of the spinal cord. The translated legend reads "Shows the Spinal Marrow whole taken out of its bony Den, and half taken from the Membrane cloathing it". The letter B signifies "The Spinal Artery seen to descend through the whole marrow which however is made up of Arteries, brought into it from between several joyntings of the Vertebrae".

opened in the midline and reflected. The appearances are those of the spinal cord of a human or animal fetus, the nerve roots of which enter and exit almost transversely through the dural sleeves. The 13a table contains five important parts. Figure 12.2 of table 13 is the famous illustration showing the origin of the anterior spinal artery from tributaries of both vertebral arteries. This figure shows a considerable understanding of the anatomical complexity of the spinal cord

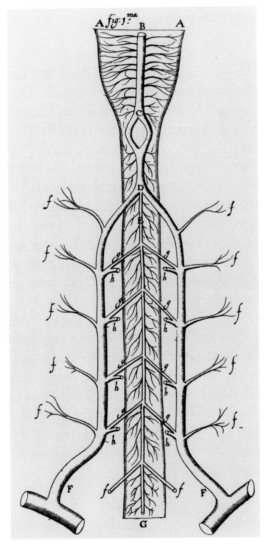

Figure 12.2 Table XIII, figure 1, from Willis' Cerebri Anatome (1664). The figure shows the vertebral arteries and their branches forming the anterior spinal artery. The translated legend reads "Shows the branching forth of the Vertebral Artery reaching out on both sides into the superior parts of the Spinal Marrow". The letter *D* signifies "The first joyning together of the Vertebral Artery above the spinal Marrow, from which place the spinal Artery descends. "The letter *g* represents "Shoots sent in the Spinal Marrow which joyn together from either side in the Spinal Marrow nigh the several joynings of the Vertebrae". The letters *f* are given as "Two Arteries sent down from the Aorta into the Spine".

vasculature. A modern criticism would be that the anterior spinal cord artery and its tributaries are shown as regular structures with equal tributaries, whereas they are irregular with grossly differing size of the arterial tributary vessels. Figure 12.2 also shows the spinal veins, the upper part of which are shown to drain into the jugular veins. Another of Willis' figures shows the posterior aspect of spinal arteries throughout the whole extent of the cord, and the plexus of arterial tributaries are indicated. Again the error is in portraying them as regular mathematically arranged structures.

The Book

The work referred to above was published in a book that has attained great fame, and some words about its production are of interest. The text was written by Willis and the drawings are by Richard Lower and Christopher Wren, possibly with additions by Willis and others. Probably completed in 1663, the work was first published in 1664. The first edition was in quarto, was published by John Martyn and James Allestry, who used the printer James Fletcher of London for the quarto edition, and Thomas Roycroft for a cheaper octavo edition, also produced in 1664. Fifteen plates were included in the first edition, and the engraver was probably David Loggan, who lived near Oxford at that time and subsequently became engraver to Oxford University. Plates 12 and 13 are those with the illustrations of the blood supply of the spinal cord, but these are the last two plates, as two unnumbered plates were inserted following plates 6 and 8.

Following the first two London editions, there were several Amsterdam editions, beginning with one also issued in 1664. The contemporary importance of the work is emphasized by the number of editions that followed, and these have been analyzed by H. R. Denham of the Wellcome Historical Medical Library. The only English translation is Samuel Pordage's, first published in London in 1681 in a collected work entitled *The Remaining Medical Works of Dr. Thomas Willis*. This is now accessible in a facsimilie edition published by the McGill University Press in 1965 and edited by William Feindel. This modern work is in two volumes, and the first volume contains valuable notes by Feindel on Willis, his work and his medical and scientific colleagues.

Thomas Willis' Successors

The publication of the work described above on the anatomy of the spinal cord vessels, was followed by several similar accounts. Most of these accounts, until that of von Haller, were derived from Willis.

Gerard Blasius (1626-1692) knew the works of Thomas Willis well and reedited them for publication in Amsterdam. His own book *Anatome Medullae Spinalis, et Nervorum* was published in 1666 and contains the same plate that appeared in Willis' book. Although he made his own observations on the spinal

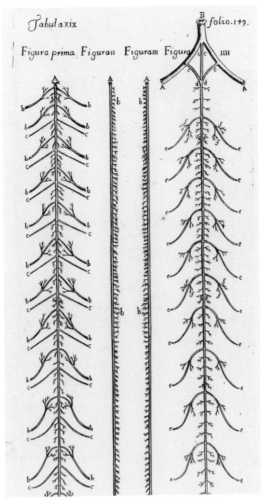

Figure 12.3 Tabula XIX, folio 149 Vieussens' *Nevrographia universalis* (1684), Lugdum, Joannen Certe. The figures show the anterior (right) and posterior (left) spinal arteries.

cord vessels, he is chiefly known for his distinction of the anterior and posterior nerve roots and the gray matter from the white matter of the spinal cord. Molinetti, in his work *Dissertationes anatomico-pathologicae* in 1675, described the union of two spinal branches of the vertebral arteries into one "rete mirabile", which he called the spinal artery. He showed how several small branches of the vertebral artery and the descending aorta contribute to the spinal artery.

Vieussens (1684) studied the vascular supply of the spinal cord. He produced many drawings of his findings, and these showed the anterior spinal artery beginning as a union of three tributaries, one from each vertebral artery and one from the basilar artery. He drew the anterior spinal artery as a regular longitudinal structure with regular tributaries accompanying each spinal nerve root and in this way perpetuated the error of Willis. He also studied the vessels of the posterior

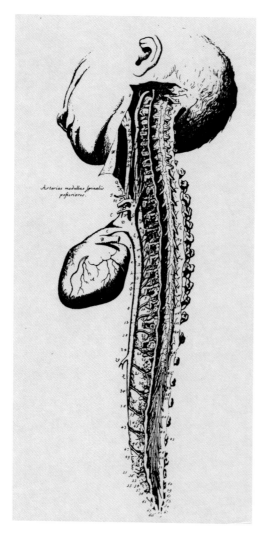

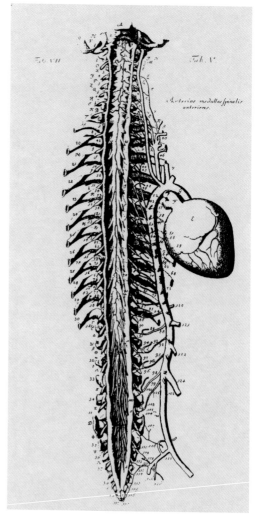

Figure 12.4 Tabula IV from *Haller's Icinum Anatomicarum Corporis Humani* (1754), Gottingen. The figure shows a drawing of a dissected and injected specimen displaying the anterior spinal arteries.

Figure 12.5 Tabula V from *Haller's Icinum Anatomicarum Corporis Humani* (1754), Gottingen. The figure shows a drawing of a dissected and injected specimen displaying the posterior spinal arteries.

aspect of the spinal cord and showed how the cephalic origin of these was from a vessel on each side arising from a cerebellar artery. He drew the posterior spinal arteries as a single vessel throughout most of their course with regular tributaries accompanying each posterior nerve root. In this regular reinforcement of the spinal cord blood supply of the posterior spinal artery, Vieussens made errors similar to those of Willis.

I shall close this chapter with a note on the work of Albrecht von Haller (1708-1777). Albrecht von Haller was an admirer of Willis and first used the phrase "circle of Willis." He studied with great care the spinal cord vascular supply, making drawings remarkable in quality and accuracy (see Figures 12.4 & 12.5). Although he undoubtedly knew of the works of Thomas Willis, his studies show no evidence of following earlier errors and, with his diagrams we arrive at the understanding of the spinal cord blood supply that we have today.

ACKNOWLEDGEMENT

I wish to acknowledge the administrators of the Bodleian Library, Oxford, England, for the use of the reproductions of some of the illustrations that appear in this chapter.

William Petty: Oxford Anatomist and Physician

The fame of Sir William Petty (1623-1687) – scientist, inventor, ship designer, surveyor, cartographer, statistician, demographer, and political economist –, has eclipsed his earlier career in anatomy and medicine, yet his few years in Oxford provide evidence of his genius in these subjects (Figure 13.1). Abundant records survive of Petty, notably the 'Petty Papers' and his published correspondence with Sir Robert Southwell.[1][2][3] John Evelyn, John Aubrey, and Samuel Pepys, knew Petty well, and with Anthony Wood, were his contemporary biographers.[4][5][6][7]

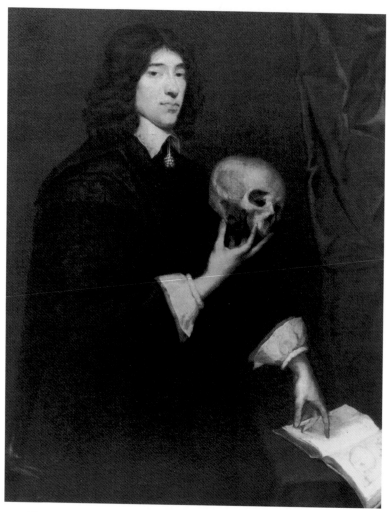

Figure 13.1 Sir William Petty. From a painting by Isaac Fuller in the National Portrait Gallery, London, and reproduced by permission.

His life was researched by a descendant, Lord Edmond Fitzmaurice, who reproduces the autobiography in Petty's will.[8] More recent biographies are by Strauss, Sharp, and Dale.[9][10][11] None of these accounts emphasises the achievements of Petty in anatomy and medicine, and what follows draws additionally from the archives of the University of Oxford, and the 'Petty Papers', formerly at Bowood House.

Birth and Early Life

William Petty came from a family of dyers in Romsey, Hampshire, and his father, Anthony, and his grandfather, John, occupied a house in Church street, which, destroyed by fire in 1826, is now replaced by the buildings numbered 28-32. Born on May 26th, 1623, William was the third child of Frances; there were to be six children, of whom only William and a younger sister, Dorothy, lived to have issue. Accounts of William describe a hyperactive, inventive child, skilled in the crafts of blacksmiths, instrument makers, watchmakers, and carpenters. By the age of twelve he was competent in Latin, and commencing Greek; his schoolmaster was a Mr King. Petty had a remarkable memory and, according to Aubrey, could 'at first hearing remember fifty nonsensical and incoherent words, and not only repeat them readily forwards and backwards, but also readily which was the 3rd, 19th, 37th, *etc.*'. At the age of about fourteen he served as a cabin boy in a small merchant ship trading with France and, '...having been 10/12 at sea, I broak my leg, and was turned ashore strangely visited by many, by ye name of "*le petit Matelot Anglois qui parle Latin et Grec*"...'.[12] His salvors in Normandy were kind and he supported himself by modest trading – in which he was precociously proficient – paying 'La Grande Jane', the farrier's wife, who set his fracture, and the apothecary who made his crutches. Becoming casually acquainted with the pupils of the Jesuit College of La Fleche in Caen, the elders learnt of his classical education, and offered him tuition in the College. Here he studied mathematics to a proficiency that became apparent later in his career of applied statistics, commanding:

> the Latin, Greek, and French tongue; the whole body of common arithmetic, the practical geometry and astronomy; conducing to navigation, dialling &c. ... preferred me to the King's Navy.[13]

But the duration of his service in the Royal Navy was short; when on lookout, his extreme shortsightedness had hazarded the ship, and a naval career for Petty was never likely.

Medical Education in Holland and France

Petty's father, Anthony, died in 1644, and was buried at Romsey.[14] Petty returned home to arrange the business and finances of the family, but already had turned to a career in medicine. In 1643: '...when the civil war betwixt the King and Parliament grew hatt, I ...vigourously followed my studies, especially that of

medicine, att Utretch, Leydon, Amsterdam, and Paris...'.[15] He matriculated as a
student of medicine at the University of Leiden on May 26th, 1644, his twenty first
birthday, and in the previous year had enrolled at Utrecht.[16] He also attended a
seven month practical course in chemistry in Holland.[17] By November 1645 he was
in Paris, bearing letters of recommendation to Hobbes from John Pell, of
Cambridge, who, since 1643, had been professor of mathematics in Amsterdam.
Petty studied anatomy with Hobbes, and gained introduction to the circle of
mathematicians and philosophers in Paris, centred on Friar Marin Mersenne.[18]
Hobbes had left England in 1640, when the Long Parliament impeached Strafford
and Laud. The medical, anatomical and scientific teaching that Petty received in
the Low Countries and Paris was superior to that available in England, even before
the disturbance of the conflict between King and Parliament. Petty was a
peripatetic student, sampling tuition in several medical schools, but in none,
seemingly, was a doctorate of medicine conferred on him. After completing his
medical studies he '...returned to Rinsey, where I was born, bringing back with me
my brother Anthony, whom I had bred...'.[19] Having arranged the business of his
late father, he removed to London, to medical studies and practice, anatomy
teaching, and scientific pursuits. Anthony had died and Petty wrote to his cousin,
John, offering him work: 'If I undertake anything in Chymistry or Anatomy,
wheereupon I shall need your assistance...'.[20]

Oxford and Brasenose College

Petty was intruded into Oxford by parliamentary bias: 'he sided with the people
then in authority', says Wood. He had no strong religious convictions and Aubrey
relates how 'He can be an excellent droll (if he haz a mind to it) and will preach
extempore incomparably, either the Presbyterian way, Independent, Cappucin frier,
or Jesuite.'[21] Politically he was for Parliament, although, in his own interest and,
preferring to complete his education, he was abroad for most of the Civil War. The
Battle of Naseby, in June, 1645, ended hope of a military victory for Charles, and
on June 24th, 1646, Oxford surrendered to the parliamentarians, who soon
required political changes in the University. Initially a lenient conversion was
attempted – even eloquent puritan preaching – but stubborn opposition of the
dons brought sterner measures, compelled by the Parliamentary Visitors,
appointed in May, 1647. The Vice-Chancellor and the Proctors were removed
from office, college heads were ejected and dons deprived of fellowships. Brasenose
was one of many colleges resisting the Visitors, who proceeded to replace Principal
Radcliffe with Daniel Greenwood, and, out of sixteen fellows, thirteen were retired
or ejected, as were several undergraduates. This purge was the background to
Petty's arrival in Oxford in 1648. John Owen and Thomas Goodwin, formerly
chaplains to Cromwell, are thought to have nominated Petty for his advancement
in Oxford. On March 7th, 1649/50, he obtained his MD.[22] In December 1650, he

was appointed a fellow of Brasenose College, displacing Nathaniel Hoyle ; and in 1650 he was elected vice-principal of the College.[23] Petty also had friends in London for, on June 25th, 1650, he was admitted a Candidate of the College of Physicians.[24] In February, 1650 he succeeded Richard Knight as Professor of Music at Gresham College – 'by the interest of his dear friend capt. Joh. Graunt.' writes Wood.[25][26]

Tomlins Readership in Anatomy [27][28]

In 1624, Richard Tomlins, of the City of Westminster did 'found constitute and ordayne an Anatomye Lector to bee for ever read and performed in the said Vniversitie...'. It was noted that 'there is as yet in neither of the Universities of this Kingdome ...any such Anotomy Lecture founded or established...'. As the first Reader, Tomlins did 'nominate and make special choyce of his worthy frend Thomas Clayton', who was Regius Professor of Medicine. Clayton's lectures were based on readings from Galen, as he seems not to have studied outside Oxford.[29] Thomas Clayton died in 1647 and was succeeded as Regius by his son, Thomas, who also became Reader in Anatomy, for which, according to Wood, he was unfitted 'being posses'd with a timorous and effeminate Humour, could never endure the sight of a mangled or bloody body.'[30] Petty deputised for Thomas Clayton as lecturer in anatomy, but on January 1st, 1650/1651, replaced him: '*in Lectura Anatomina ex fundatio Rich Tomkins, Giul. Petty*'.[31] He was also appointed Professor of Public Anatomy. This began systematic teaching of modern anatomy in Oxford.

Anatomy in Oxford

Before Petty, anatomy was taught in Oxford by reading in Latin from a raised throne, viewing a human dissection performed by a surgeon. Galen's works were specified in the statutes, but more appropriate was the dissecting manual of Mundinus, first published in 1316. Whilst Oxford had attracted several modern anatomists – notably William Harvey –, the tuition before Petty was of classical anatomy. Anatomical teaching was directed by the Laudian Statutes of the Carolinan Code, a restatement of existing statutes, made in 1638 by the authority of Archbishop Laud.[32] Medical students had to see two anatomical dissections before obtaining the BA, and observe others before obtaining the DM. Additional to the statutes dating from 1564/5, those of the 1624 Tomlin's benefaction, specified details.[33] The Reader was commanded:

> 2. ...every Springe immediately after the ...Lent Assisses for the County of Oxon., upon the procuring of a Sounde body of one of the Executed persons ...cause the said body to bee prepared and dissected by a skilfull Chirurgian : And hee the said Reader shall publiquely shewe, teach and deliver the Scituation, Nature, Vse and office, of the partes of the body in ffoure distinct Lectures...

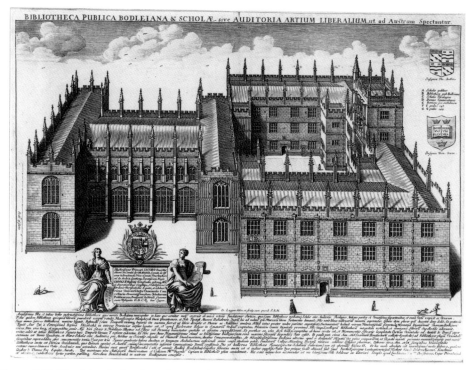

Figure 13.2 The Schools Quadrangle, seen from the south, from Loggan's Oxonia illustrata, 1675

These four lectures or 'meetings' were specified in the Tomlins statute:

> 3. The next Morning ...the Reader with the Chirurgian standing by him (for the severing lyfting vp and shewing of the partes) shall for two hourses space shewe the Scituation, Nature, Vse and office of the partes commonly called Naturall videlicet Liver Spleene Stomake Guttes &.

The dissections and lectures occupied this and the succeeding day for:

> 4. The same day in the afternoone the Reader ...shall (in two houres) further deliver and teach the Scituation Nature and office of the same Naturall partes.

> 5. The next morning . . . The Reader shall deliver publiquely (in two houres as aforesaid) the Scituation Nature and office of the partes commonly called Vitall videlicet Hart Lunges &.

> 6. The same day after noone ...the Reader shall ...shew and teach the Scituation Nature and Office of the Animal partes and faculties videlicet the Brayne &.

Anatomy was taught twice-yearly over two days by these demonstrations of human dissection, which were popular public events, not confined to medical students. They originally took place in the Anatomy School, which can be seen in Loggan's engraving (Figure 13.2) as the first three windows on the left of the first floor of the elevation in the forefront, an area now within the Lower Reading

Room of the Bodleian Library.   Human dissection was a race against decomposition and in the summer term was not attempted. The Reader was paid 'Twenty fyve pounds yearely' and from this sum paid his surgeon £3 for each dissection and, to others, £ 2 for the transport and 'decent buriall of the body and all necessaries thervnto belonging'. In the Michaelmas term the Reader lectured on 'the Sceleton or History of the bones with theire Scituation Nature and Office'.

Petty as Anatomist

The extracts above are from the statutes of the Tomlins Reader, but what Petty taught is known from his lecture notes, many of which survive.[34] In 1646 he was

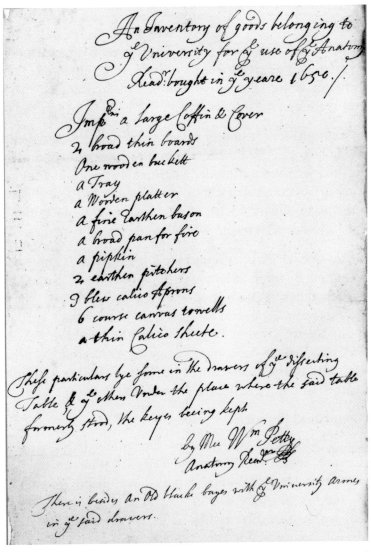

Figure 13.3 Inventory of goods required by Petty on becoming Anatomy Reader. (Reproduced, by permission, from the Oxford University Archives, SEP. L.11.Z1).

studying in Paris and he brought his '*Cursus Anatomicus*' to Oxford.[35] In 1649, as deputy to Thomas Clayton, he had given 'Six *Phisico-Medicall*' lectures.[36] His inaugural lecture as Tomlins Reader was given on March 4th 1650/1651.[37] Among the Petty Papers are several texts of his anatomy lectures. These were in Latin, but, years later, Petty lectured on anatomy to the College of Physicians in Dublin and this text is in English.[38]

Petty discontinued *ex cathedra* lecturing from a raised throne, whilst a surgeon demonstrated the dissection. Not only did he dissect himself, but he urged his students also to study '...not by bookes but *per autopsum* the anatomy of Man, of a dog, of a cock and hen, a salmon, eele, lobster, and oyster.'[39] Comparative anatomy was recommended, particularly of small animals, – easily procured and dissected :

> Whereas if you fleece and exinterate a Ratt, or some thin animall, you may then by holding up his extended flesh against the bright sunn ...disern how the vessels ly one to the other, ...with more satisfaction then the tracing of branch after branch of greater animals.[40]

Petty's papers include three lectures in osteology, a subject required as 'the Sceleton or History of the bones ...'.[41] For tuition in osteology, human and animal bones had to be procured, and Petty compiled instructions on 'boiling bones'.[42] A list of Petty's requisites for anatomical teaching, purchased in 1650, includes a coffin, for transporting the body (Figure 13.3)[43]. '...Ye dissecting Table' and 'an old blacke [sheet] with ye University Armes ...' was inherited from his predecessors.

The 1636 charter of Charles I permitted the Tomlins Reader to demand the body of any person executed within twenty-one miles of Oxford, as the famous case of Anne Greene exemplifies. Petty gained immediate renown from the resuscitation of Anne, who, hanged and supplied for dissection in December 1650, proved to be alive.[44] The body was received at Petty's rooms, and dissection was to take place in the morning, seemingly in his rooms (Figure 13.4) Anatomical dissections were of great interest and to the scene had come Thomas Willis, Ralph Bathurst, and Henry Clerke, the last named being the Vice-Chancellor.

Medical Lectures and Practice

His doctorate in Medicine, conferred in December 1650, permitted clinical practice in Oxford, which complemented Petty's lectures in medicine. He also lectured on chemistry, a favorite subject, studied in Holland. Knowledge of syphilis was essential, and his '*de Arthridide et Lue Venera...*' dated 1646, and marked 'Paris Oxford', arose from his studies in Paris.[45] Another lecture on '*De Lue Venera*' survives.[46] The scale of his practice is evident from notes on prescriptions, herbs, purgatives, and individual clinical cases.[47] His practice included addresses in Oxford, Bath, London, Reading, and Timsbury.[48] By 1652, out of a total annual

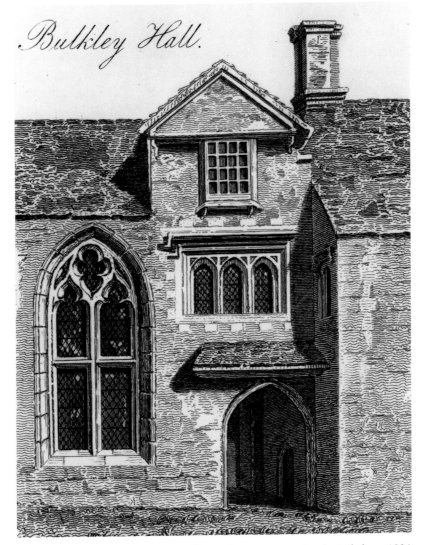

Figure 13.4 Bulkley Hall, lodgings of Petty. From an engraving by J Skelton, 1821.

income of £ 800, his medical work earned £ 280.[49] Petty's reputation was high in the College of Physicians of London, but his other interests and his long periods in Ireland precluded regular attendance, and according to Munk, 'His life affords but few incidents of a medical character…'.[50] He was elected a fellow in July 1655, but, being away in Ireland, was not admitted till June 1658. Whilst Petty practised some medicine throughout most of his career, in later years, he regretted his preoccupation with other interests, writing in 1686:

> …I could Anno 1656 have returned into England and been at the top of practice in Oliver's Court, when Dr Willis was casting waters at Abingdon Markett and the Cock Lowre [Richard Lower] but an egge.[51]

Science and the Royal Society

Petty's support of the Royal Society was important in its foundation. In London he had been admitted to several 'clubbs of the virtuosi', and on arriving in Oxford, he found old colleagues and was joined by others. Aubrey wrote: '…about these times experimental philosophy first budded there and was first cultivated by these vertuosi in that darke time…', and named Ralph Bathurst, John Wilkins, Seth Ward, Robert Wood, and Thomas Willis, as Petty's associates. The complex antecedents of the Royal Society have been much researched, and I quote only from the account of Birch.[52] In 1648 and 1649 some London virtuosi moved to Oxford, notably Dr Wilkins to become warden of Wadham in April 1648, Dr Wallis, to the chair of Geometry in June 1649, and Dr Goddard to be warden of Merton in December 1651. These with Seth Ward in the chair of Astronomy from 1649, and Thomas Willis, exceptionally a Royalist, were the close colleagues who met : '…at first in Dr Petty's lodgings, in the house of an apothecary, for the convenience of inspecting drugs…', and after '…his departure in September 1652 to Ireland, they met …at Dr Wilkin's apartments in Wadham College…'. Subsequently Petty was a founder of the Royal Society and an enthusiastic attender. However his science, for example in physics and chemistry, never equalled others, such as Boyle, as a meeting on January 2, 1660/1661 compares. Boyle was requested to '…bring in his cylinder, and to shew . . . his experiment of the air…', whilst Petty's subject was '…the history of the building of ships…'.[53] But, Petty regularly attended and contributed – in a lively manner. Aubrey relates an amusing discussion of a patron saint for the Society, when Petty advanced Saint Thomas, for his insistence of proof.

Ireland, Fame, and Fortune

In April 1651 the Visitors granted Petty two years leave of absence from Oxford with an annual allowance of £30, an exceptional benefit, but Petty was in favour with the Parliamentarians, who controlled the University, with Cromwell as Chancellor. Scarcely had this leave begun, when he was made physician to the army in Ireland and to the person and family of the Lieutenant-General. In Ireland, Petty soon enlarged his activities, by surveying the country, displacing Benjamin Worsley, whose survey he decided was 'most insufficiently and absurdly managed'. Petty's subsequent complex career was inextricably tied to Ireland, where he made his fame and fortune, surviving the restoration and being knighted in 1661. Petty's fame in statistics and political economy endures, but his career in medicine and several other fields, including political advancement, fell short of lasting achievement. The shrewd opinion of Charles II was: 'the man will not be contented to be excellent, but is still ayming at impossible things'.[54]

ACKNOWLEDGEMENT

I thank the staff of the Bodleian Library for their continuing assistance and for the use of their microfilm of the Petty Papers. I am indebted to the Lansdowne family and specifically to the Earl of Shelburne in permitting the use of these manuscripts.

NOTES AND REFERENCES

1 Slatter MD. *Calendar of Literary and Personal Papers of Sir William Petty*. Lists the 'Petty Papers' [PP], now held in the British Library, but also on microfilm. Bodleian Library *MSS Film 1944-59*. The medical papers are in vol. 3.

2 Lansdowne, Marquis of. *The Petty Papers* [Henceforth Lans. TPP]. London : Constable, 1927.

3 Lansdowne, Marquis of. *The Petty-Southwell Correspondence*. [Henceforth Lans. PSC] London: Constable, 1928.

4 Evelyn J. *The Diary of John Evelyn*. Vols 1-3. Edited by A. Dobson. London: Macmillan, 1906, several entries.

5 Aubrey J. *Brief Lives*. Edited by A. Clark. Oxford: Clarendon Press, 1898 : 2, 139-50.

6 Pepys S. *The Diary of Samuel Pepys*. Vols 1-8. Edited by H.B. Wheatley. London: Bell & Sons, 1942, several entries.

7 Wood A. *Athenae Oxonienses*. Vols 1-4. Edited by P. Bliss. London: Many Publishers, 1813, 2, 119-20, 2, 156, 3, 1120, and 4, 214-20.

8 Fitzmaurice, Lord Edmond. *The Life of Sir William Petty*. London: John Murray, 1895 [Henceforth Fitz]. Appendix 11 reproduces the will, dated 2.5.1685, Court of Probate in Ireland.

9 Strauss E. *Sir William Petty, Portrait of a Genius*. London: Bodley Head, 1954.

10 Sharp GL. *Sir William Petty and some aspects of Seventeenth Century Natural Philosophy*. Oxford : D.Phil Thesis, University of Oxford, 1976.

11 Dale PG. *Sir W. P. of Romsey*. Romsey: LTVAS Group, 1987.

12 *Lans. PSC*, 216-7. Letter to Sir R. Southwell, July 14, 1686.

13 *Lans. PSC*, 216-7.

14 Romsey Parish Reg. Burial on 14.7.1644.

15 Fitz., 319.

16 Innes Smith RW. *English-Speaking Students of Medicine at the University of Leyden*. Edinburgh & London : Oliver and Boyd, 1932, 181.

17 Fitz., 317.

18 *Dictionary of National Biography*. London: Smith, Elder & Co, 1908, 11, 931-9.

19 Fitz., 319.

20 Fitz., 13-15.

21 Aubrey, 2, 143.

22 *Univ. Oxon. Arch*. Cong. Reg. 1648-59, f 182r.

23 Wood, 4, 215.

24 Munk W. *The Roll of The Royal College of Physicians of London*. 2nd. ed. London: Published by the College, 1878, 271.

25 Wood, 4, 213.

[26] Ward J. *The Lives of the Professors of Gresham College.* London: Printed by John Moore, 1740, 217-27.

[27] Ward GRM. *Translation of Oxford University Statutes.* London: Pickering, 1845.

[28] Gibson S., Editor. *Statuta antiqua universalis oxoniensis.* Oxford: Clarendon Press, 1931.

[29] Clark A. *Register of the University of Oxford.* Oxford: Clarendon Press, 1888, 2, 3, 184.

[30] Wood, 4, 215.

[31] *Univ. Oxon Arch.* Conv. Reg. 1647-1659, 31.12.1650, 124.

[32] Griffiths J. *Statutes of the University of Oxford codified in the year 1638 under the authority of Archbisop Laud.* Oxford: Clarendon Press, 1888, 125-127.

[33] Gibson, 551-5, and Griffiths, 258-61.

[34] *PP.* The medical papers are grouped 1-31 in Vol 3.

[35] Fitz., 317, 1646, Paris and Oxford.

[36] Fitz., 317, 1649, Oxford.

[37] *PP.* 3, 27.

[38] *PP.* 3, 25. Reproduced in Lans. TPP, 171-179.

[39] Lands. TPP, 169.

[40] Lands. TPP, 178.

[41] Fitz., Appendix 1, 1650, London.

[42] *PP.* 3, 23.

[43] *Univ. Oxon Arch.*, SEP. L ii, 21.

[44] Hughes JT. 'Miraculous deliverance of Anne Green: an Oxford case of resuscitation in the seventeenth century', *British Medical Journal*, 285 (1982), 1702-1703. Lists references.

[45] Fitz., 317, 1646, Paris and Oxford.

[46] *PP.* 3, 19.

[47] *PP.* vol. 3, 6, 8, 13, 17, and 21.

[48] *PP.* 3, 21.

[49] Lans. PSC, 214-5. Letter to Southwell, 13.7.1686.

[50] Munk, 271.

[51] Lans. PSC, 214-5.

[52] Birch T. *The History of the Royal Society of London.* London: A Millar, 1755, 1, 1-3.

"Alas Poor Yorick"! : the Death of Laurence Sterne

Summary: The life and death of Laurence Sterne are examined. Sterne's body was taken from his grave and soon after appeared for dissection in Cambridge. The teaching of anatomy, the activities of body snatchers and the passage of the 1832 Anatomy Act are reviewed.

The publication in London (1760) of the first two parts of *Tristram Shandy* transformed Laurence Sterne (1713-1768) (Figure 14.1) from an obscure Yorkshire clergyman into a literary figure acclaimed as a genius and given the sobriquet 'Yorick'.[1] Sterne shared the fate of Shakespeare's Yorick - his grave was disturbed, but by robbers seeking a body for anatomical dissection. Written records of this trade are scarce – resurrectionists preferred oral communication.

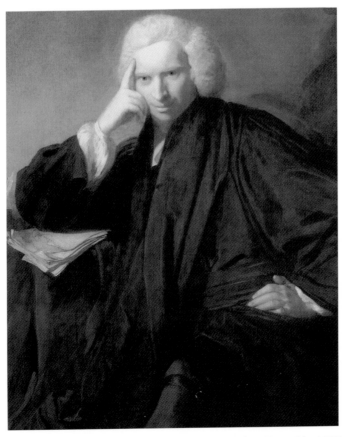

Figure 14.1 The 'Landscape' portrait of Laurence Sterne by Sir Joshua Reynolds, 1760. (Reproduced by permission of the National Portrait Gallery, NPG 5019.)

Contemporary records describe Sterne's illness, his last days, and the grim sequence of his death, burial, resurrection, and dissection. The activities of the 'body snatchers' or 'resurrectionists', the anatomists who required this trade, and the 1832 Anatomy Act are described.

Sterne's life before Tristram Shandy

Sterne has many biographers of which the most important are Fitzgerald,[2] Traill ,[3] Cross,[4] and Cash.[5] Sterne's letters have been edited by Curtiss.[6] There is a short autobiography.[7] Of his published works, *Tristram Shandy* and *A Sentimental Journey* refer obliquely to events in his life.[8] However, his eight years after the publication of Tristram Shandy are recorded in greater detail than the forty-six preceding years.

Sterne's father was Roger Sterne, a Lieutenant in the 34th Regiment of Foot, who had married an Agnes Herbert, the daughter of a quartermaster. Laurence was the second child, born on 24 November 1713 in Clonmel, Ireland, to which the regiment had returned from Dunkirk after the Peace of Utrecht. The family was consumptive and, of six children, only the three eldest survived infancy. Laurence lived ten years in several army barracks interspersed by journeys on land, and voyages by sea, between England and Ireland. At the age of ten he was fortunate to be sent to school in Halifax, staying with a wealthy uncle.[9]

After the death of his father in 1731 and his uncle in 1732, his cousin, Richard, assisted Laurence to study classics and divinity at Jesus College, Cambridge. In 1737 he graduated BA and was ordained into the Church of England as a deacon. His career was advanced by his uncle, Dr Jacques Sterne, Archdeacon of Cleveland and Precentor of York Minster. Ordained priest in 1738, Sterne received the living of Sutton-on-the-Forest, and six years later added the neighbouring living of Stillington. In 1741 he married Elizabeth Lumley, who bore Sterne two daughters but only Lydia, born in 1747, survived. For twenty two years Sterne lived the obscure life of a country parson. His sermons interested his congregations, but apart from some journalism, supporting the Whigs, he was not noticed elsewhere.

Fame in London and Paris

In 1760, the success of the first two volumes of *Tristram Shandy* changed Sterne's life. The reviewer in the *London Magazine* of February was ecstatic, and, in March, Sterne journeyed to London, where he was invited everywhere, received many favours, and, by 11 March, was installed in rooms in Pall Mall

> 'the genteelest in Town, are full of the greatest Company. I dined these 2 days with 2 ladies of the bedchamber; then with Ld Rockingham, Ld Edgecomb, Lord Winchelsea, Lord Littelton, a Bishop &, &'. [10]

Two weeks after Sterne arrived in London, Lord Fauconberg of Newburgh Prior, Coxwold offered him the living of Coxwold, and his house there, to be called

'Shandy Hall', became Sterne's residence in Yorkshire. David Garrick was an early acquaintance and introduced Sterne to Bishop Warburton (of Gloucester), a prominent literary figure in London, and Warburton, who had described Sterne as 'the English Rabelais', gave Sterne several books and a purse of gold.[11] Such was Sterne's fame that on 20 March he attended the studio of Joshua Reynolds for the first of eight sittings for his portrait. (Figure 14.1) The Marquis of Rockingham – leader of the Yorkshire Whigs and Lord Lieutenant of the North and West Ridings - took Sterne to Windsor Castle on May 6 to witness his installation as Knight of the Garter.[12]

In May 1760 Sterne returned to his family in York and took them to his new living in Coxwold, began the publication of his sermons, and resumed the writing of *Tristram Shandy*, of which parts III and IV appeared in Janaury 1761, and parts VII and VIII in December 1761. These many activities throughout summer and autumn undermined Sterne's health, deciding him to move to France. He arrived in Paris in January 1762, to a reception which exceeded that of London: '('tis *comme a Londres*) ...a fortnight's dinners and suppers on my hands'.[13] Amongst intellectuals he made friends, but soon tired of the society in the salons of Paris. His health further deteriorated and in July he removed with his wife and daughter to Toulouse,[14] then to Montpellier.[15] But by 1764 France displeased: '...for I am heartily tired of it – that insipidity there is in French characters has disgusted your friend Yorick.'[16] Moreover he had, tired by an unfortunate riding experience, become ill, being in bed ten days in 'scuffle with death'. He returned to England, having established his wife and daughter in Montauban. In 1765 he made a journey through France and Italy, returning in 1766.

Sterne now was the incumbent at Coxwold, but in London he took rooms on the first floor of a house in Old Bond Street, the third on the left from Picadilly and now No 48.[17] His widowed landlady was Mrs Fourmantel who made silken bags in which gentlemen, including the king, tied their back hair. Here he lived in comfort, entertained, and was constantly visited. He published his sermons and the remaining seven volumes of *Tristram Shandy*, and, shortly before his death, *A Sentimental Journey*.

Sterne's tuberculosis

Laurence's mother suffered from pulmonary tuberculosis, and generalised tuberculosis was the probable cause of the early death of his brothers and sisters, save one who died of smallpox. His father died of a fever contracted in Port Antonio, Trinidad, but had not recovered from a duelling wound through his chest – he also might have been consumptive. In 1641, Sterne married Elizabeth Lumley, who herself had made an imperfect recovery from tuberculosis. Their first child died the day after birth, the second, Lydia, was tuberculous. Sterne was ill from childhood, and at Cambridge, experienced a major haemoptysis.[18] His illness was chronic fibro-caseous pulmonary tuberculosis.[19] His adult life was a battle with tuberculosis, improved by rest and tranquillity, but worsened by the work of writing and the indulgences of society in London. His letters are punctuated by many reports of haemoptysis, but one episode was a painful testicular swelling, thought by his physicians to be syphilitic, and treated with courses of mercury.[20] Syphilitic gumma are usually painless, and this complication may have been a tuberculous abscess. Sterne also complained of lassitude and fatigue, which frequently confined him to bed. His writing and social engagements continued but he was aware that 'if I am rash enough to risk the Winter in London, I shall never see another Spring.'[21]

Sterne's Death

Before *A Sentimental Journey* was published on 27 February 1768, Sterne had been busy with proofs and obtaining advance copies from the bindery for his friends. By March he was ill, in bed, and unable to sit for Sir Joshua Reynolds on the 9th. By March 15, Sterne was very ill, and writing to Mrs James – his last letter – he had to 'rest his hand a dozen times'. He was; 'at death's door this week with pleurisy – I was bled three times on Thursday, and blister'd on Friday...' Aware of his illness and that of his wife he commended his daughter to Mrs James should 'my child want a mother'.[22] Sterne died at four in the afternoon of Friday, March

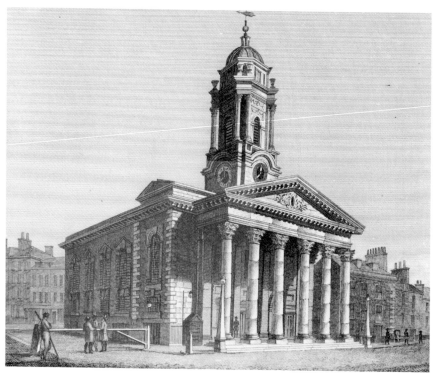

Figure 14.2 Engraving of St George's, Hanover Square. (Author's collection.)

18, 1768. None of his family were around him, and except for his landlady and a nurse, only one person – John Macdonald – witnessed his death. Macdonald was the servant of John Craufurd, who was entertaining at dinner a great company, including the Dukes of Grafton and Roxburgh, the Earls of March and Ossory and Mr David Garrick. The guests enquired after Sterne's health, and Macdonald was sent to report, arriving five minutes before Sterne died.[23]

The funeral service took place on Tuesday, March 22 at St George's Church, Hanover Square (Figure 14.2).[24] Officiating was the rector, the Rev. Dr Charles Moss, who had recently become the Bishop of St David's.[25] Probably many of his London friends attended, but no record survives of the numbers present. Notices stressed the incongruity of his fame compared with his lonely death, remarking on his poverty and desertion by his friends and relatives – the sequence of a 'Rake's Progress'. The truth is different. He lived beyond his income, but *A Sentimental Journey* had now been published and its sale promised funds. He was living, not in a garret, but in a fashionable part of London and seen by many friends until visits were prevented by his illness. On the night he died, he was remembered at an elegant party nearby, where he would have been welcome, if well. He was on indifferent terms with his wife who, herself ill with tuberculosis, was absent from his deathbed and funeral, as was his daughter.

Sterne's burial, resurrection, and anatomical dissection

The burial-ground was some way from the church, and only two mourners are known to have attended: Thomas Becket, Sterne's bookseller, and Samuel Salt, his lawyer. His bookseller was concerned with *A Sentimental Journey*, and possibly unpublished manuscripts. His lawyer may have been involved with an agreement concerning his wife and daughter. His many London friends might not have known of his lonely burial, due to the absence of his family and Yorkshire friends. Hall-Stevenson, a friend since Cambridge, was absent, but, an atheist, did not attend church services.

The absence of mourners alerted the body-snatchers, who removed the body on the night of Thursday, March 24.[26] They were familiar with this burial-ground (Figure 14.3) which in November 1767 had been robbed of several bodies.[27] It was acquired from Sir Richard Grovenor in 1725, and George Clinch described it in 1892 as:

> situated just off Oxford Street, near the Marble Arch, and between Albion Street and Stanhope Street. It is a beautifully quiet and secluded area, almost entirely enclosed by tall houses, well wooded …and ornamented with some borders of old-fashioned flowers [28]

From about 1923 to 1939 the churchyard was used as the archery ground of the Royal Toxophilite Society. After World War 2 it became the block of flats

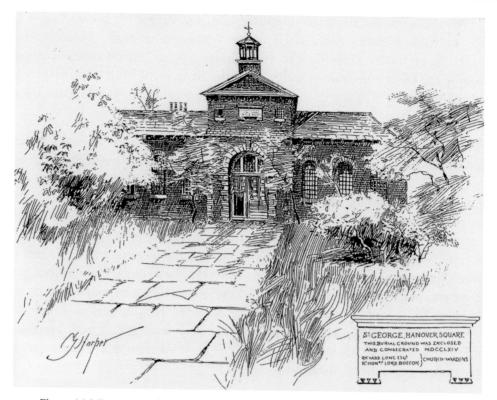

Figure 14.3 Engraving of the burial ground of St George's, Hanover Square, London. In: Clinch G. History of Mayfair and Belgravia, 1892, facing p. 52. (reproduced by permission of the Bodleian Library, University of Oxford, shelfmark G A Lond° 176.)

known as St George's Fields. A small area remains as a garden with tombstones leaning against the walls, and can be entered from Albion Street, but is private, belonging to Hyde Park Nursery School.[29]

Sterne's body was stolen on March 24th and soon after appeared for dissection in Cambridge, of which there are several accounts. The incident was reported in the *Public Advertiser*.[30] Isaac Reed at Cambridge wrote in 1787: 'the body of Mr. Sterne had been sent down to Cambridge and was anatomized'.[31] Willis's *Current Notes* quotes Edmond Malone: 'A gentleman who was present at the dissection recognized Sterne's face the moment he saw the body.'[32] Of historians of Cambridge, Professor Macalister,[33] and Sir Humprey Rolleston[34] believed the account related above. The subsequent movements of Sterne's body are less certain but its prompt return to London for reburial is likely. Subsequently two Freemasons unrelated to the family erected a gravestone, near the place of reburial, the inscription of which had several inaccuracies.[35] In 1893 a footstone and a border rail were erected by Captain F.H. Carrol of Mundiff, County Wicklow, owner of Woodhouse in Halifax, and a distant relative of Richard, cousin of Sterne.[36]

In recent times the remains of Sterne were moved to Coxwold, Yorkshire.[37] Before the block of flats were erected, Kenneth Monkman, secretary of the Laurence Sterne Trust, arranged for a search of the burial ground and the removal of Sterne's remains, which was done on 4 June 1969. Amongst the bones recovered was a skull, the crown of which had been removed, evidence of an anatomical examination. This, with other bones, thought to be related, were interred on the south side of the churchyard of St Michael's Coxwold on 8 June, 1969.

The teaching of anatomy by human dissection

Modern teaching of anatomy began in Bologna when Mondinus (Mondino de'Luzzi, 1270-1326) began public dissections of the human body in 1315.[38] His textbook of anatomical dissection – the *Anathomia* – first printed in Padua in 1478, was the first in Europe and was used for centuries in over forty editions. Mondinus was followed by Berengario de Carpi (1470-1550), Professor from 1502 to 1527, and Alessandro Achillini (1463-1512), who moved from Bologna to Padua, beginning the preeminence in Padua of anatomy. About 1539 a young Cambridge graduate – John Caius (1510-1573), of Norwich – came to Padua as Professor of Greek and, after lodging for eight months with the great Andreas Vesalius (1514-1564), turned his attention to medicine and anatomy graduating in 1540.[39] Returning to Cambridge in 1541, Caius introduced the teaching of modern anatomy to England, in the Barber-Surgeons Hall in 1546 and in Cambridge in 1547. In 1565 the bodies of two criminals or unknown strangers were granted to Caius College, Cambridge for dissection by the Regius Professor of Physic.

Teaching of anatomy in Cambridge – usually in the colleges – preceded by many years the creation of a chair of anatomy in 1707.[40] Space for the professor was provided in the Printing House, built in 1689, and, what became the first 'Anatomy House' at Cambridge, stood at the corner of Queens' Lane in Silver Street. Here for over a century anatomy was taught and bodies dissected before the students – see figure 14.4.[41] The first professor, Mr George Rolfe, neglected his duties, and, being absent for several years, his chair was declared vacant in 1728. However Rolfe taught in London as William Stukeley relates: 'went to see Courses of Anatomy with Mr. George Rolf who lived then in Chancery Lane...'.[42] Rolfe's successor, John Morgan, dissected diligently, judging by complaints of the activity of resurectionists, as Masters wrote:[43]

> the practice of digging up human bodies in the Churchyards of this town and the neighbouring Villages, and the carrying them into Colleges to be dissected...
> to the no small offence of all serious people

The problem of supply continued and later Cambridge obtained two bodies a year from London – possibly illegally – for the Professor's public dissections. The body of Sterne came to Cambridge during the tenure of Charles Collignon 1725-1785, Professor of Anatomy from 1753. Collignon, from France, was educated at

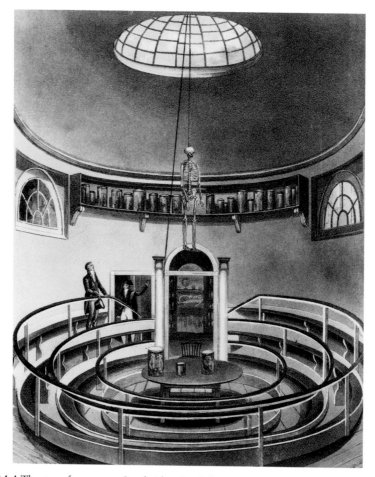

Figure 14.4 Theatre of anatomy, Cambridge. In: Ackerman R. *A History of the University of Cambridge*, 1815, facing p. 290. (Reproduced by permission of the Bodleian Library, University of Oxford, shelfmark A A b 30(2).)

Trinity College, Cambridge, graduated MB in 1749 and MD in 1754.[44] His merits as an anatomist and as a physician are doubtful and Macalister thought: 'his lectures must have been uncommonly dull for his class, which probably was a small one'.[45] Collignon's published works contain little anatomy, even those in which the title includes anatomy.[46]

The 1832 Anatomy Act

During the eighteenth century the population of London was expanding and new hospitals were added to St. Bartholomew's and St. Thomas's: Westminster (1720), Guy's (1724), St. George's (1733), the London (1740), and the Middlesex (1745).[47] In the provinces, most cities and large towns, also growing in population, opened a hospital or infirmary.[48] Addenbrookes Hospital, Cambridge was opened in 1766, and the Radcliffe Infirmary, Oxford in 1770. Expansion of existing medical schools was accompanied in London by the founding of private medical schools, in which tuition in anatomy was prominent.[49] William Cheselden,[50] a leading surgeon, taught anatomy (and physiology), in conflict with the Barber-Surgeons Company, which, with the Royal College of Physicians, claimed a monopoly on anatomical dissection. The Surgeons parted company with the Barbers in 1745 and then built their Surgeons Hall in which anatomy was taught. Already, in 1746, William Hunter had begun dissections and anatomy classes in a house in Covent Garden, joined, in 1748, by his brother John. In 1766, he bought No 16 Great Windmill Street, to be rebuilt as an anatomy school with a lecture theatre, museum, and dissecting room. The Hunter brothers were followed by other teachers in London. Anatomy teaching also expanded in the London Hospitals, in the provinces of England, and in the medical schools of Oxford, Cambridge, and, of course, of Scotland.

This expansion of anatomical teaching explains the demand for human bodies. Yet the law, from old statutes, allowed in England only a few bodies of executed criminals to be delivered to the schools of London, Oxford, and Cambridge. Body-snatching was illegal, but the law was not enforced as the removal of the body was not a crime. The disturbance of the grave was a misdemeanour, and the robbers replaced the coffin and shroud to avoid the charge of theft – a felony, with greater penalties. Resurrectionists were more at risk from the public than the authorities, who were influenced by the connivance of famous surgeons and reputable hospitals. A notable personage was Sir Astley Cooper, twice president of the Royal College of Surgeons, and an enthusiastic anatomist and dissector.[51] The surgeons at the major hospitals gave their services to patients without charge, but their philanthropy was not without self interest as they charged students for instruction, especially anatomy tuition.

When Sterne's body was stolen in 1758, the practice was common, but subsequently became much more frequent, even a systematic provision of corpses. There are many accounts.[52] Body snatchers were aided by undertakers, and the anatomists, aware of the source, shared the guilt. Poor persons dying in hospitals were frequently dissected in those or other hospitals. Bodies were stolen before the interment of an empty coffin, weighted to deceive the mourners. The ultimate crime was the murder, of poor persons without relatives or friends. Burke and Hare in Edinburgh were not resurrectionists but murdered their victims for their clients, one being the infamous Dr Knox.[53] Burke was found guilty – on the evidence of Hare – and hanged in Edinburgh in 1829, where he was publicly dissected. The London 'Burkers' were Bishop and Williams whose crimes differed from that of Burke and Hare in that they also had resurrected between 500 and 1000 corpses.[54] Bishop and Williams, convicted of the murder of three of their victims, and hanged in December 1831, probably murdered many more, possibly sixty.[55]

The response of the government to these events was not to strengthen the law against body snatching but to legalise a supply of bodies from prisons, poor law houses, and hospitals. *A Select Committee on Anatomy*, chaired by Henry Warburton,[56] had examined the problem, with much testimony from anatomists and surgeons – Astley Cooper, Benjamin Brodie, John Abernethy and many others –, and reported in 1828.[57] On 12 March 1828 Warburton introduced his first Bill for *Preventing the Unlawful Disinterment of Human Bodies, and for Regulating Schools of Anatomy*,[58] but this failed because of opposition in the Lords.[59] Ten days after the London execution of Bishop and Williams, Warburton introduced his second Anatomy Bill.[60] Debate now was less vocal, the main opponent in the Commons being Henry Hunt MP, of Spa Fields in 1816 and Peterloo in 1819. William Cobbett vehemently denounced the Bill in his Political Register.[61] Despite the eloquence of 'Orator Hunt' the Bill passed the Commons and Lords[62] and became law on 1 August 1832.[63]

An Act for Regulating Schools of Anatomy required the Home Secretary '…to appoint not fewer than Three persons to be Inspectors of Places [to be approved] where Anatomy is carried on…', and to licence members of the medical profession 'to practice Anatomy . . .'. Executors had to respect the desire not to be dissected, expressed in writing or verbally, either by the deceased or a near relative. Undertakers were prohibited from these decisions. No body was to be moved for dissection until 48 hours after death and 24 hours after permission had been given by an inspector. Bodies had to be moved in 'a decent Coffin' and after dissection 'be decently interred in consecrated ground or, in some public burial place …of the religious Persuasion', to which the deceased belonged. Prior legislation authorising the dissection of an executed criminal was repealed; important in separating anatomical dissection from punishment.

The Anatomy Act of 1832 is a milestone of anatomical teaching in Great Britain, legalising the expansion of anatomical dissection. In the subsequent year, 1832-1833, 609 bodies were provided for anatomy, 394 from parish workhouses, 135 from hospitals, 24 from prisons and hulks, 5 from asylums, and 51 from dwellings.[64] The poor dying in workhouses were the chief source.

Whilst the Act solved most of the problems of the anatomists it has been claimed that, unaware or mistrusting its safeguards, the poor feared that, if they died in poor houses or hospitals, they would not be buried but dissected.[65] The provisions in the Act quoted above indicate the safeguards included in the Act. How much care was taken by the anatomists in the eighteenth century (and subsequent years) to respect the wishes of the subjects and of their relatives is a matter for research and debate.

1832 was the year of the *Reform Act*, with modest change of the franchise, improved by the *Reform Acts* of 1867 and 1884, and the *Representation of the*

People Act in 1918. Many years would elapse before the vote was extended to the poor who were the main subjects of anatomical dissection under *The Anatomy Act* of 1832.

ACKNOWLEDGEMENTS

For much assistance, I am indebted to the staffs of the Bodleian, British, and Guildhall Libraries.

NOTES AND REFERENCES

1 Sterne L. *The Life and Opinions of Tristram Shandy, Gentleman.* York: Ann Ward, 1759 and London: Robert & James Dodsley, 1760.

2 Fitzgerald P. *The Life of Laurence Sterne*, 3rd.ed. London: Chatto and Windus, 1906

3 Traill HD. *Sterne*. London: Macmillan and Co, 1889.

4 Cross WB. *The Life and Times of Laurence Sterne*, 3rd. ed. New Haven and London: Yale University Press and Oxford University Press, 1929.

5 Cash AH. *Laurence Sterne: The Early and Middle Years*. London: Methuen, 1975; and *Laurence Sterne: The Later Years*. London: Methuen, 1986.

6 Curtiss LP. *Letters of Laurence Sterne*. Oxford: Clarendon Press, 1935.

7 First published by Lydia de Medalle. *Letters of the late Rev. Mr. Laurence Sterne, to his Most Intimate Friends*, 3 vols. 1775, 1, 1-24.

8 References are from the Letters volume of the Shakespeare Head Edition of *The Works of Laurence Sterne* (henceforth Letters), 7 vols. Oxford: Basil Blackwell, 1926.

9 Hughes JT. Laurence Sterne (1713-1768) and Hipperholme Grammar School. *Transactions of the Halifax Antiquary Society*, (Henceforth THAS) 9 (2001), 53-62.

10 Letter to Catherine de Fourmantel, undated, *Letters*, 302.

11 Letter to Catherine de Fourmantel, undated, *Letters*, 302.

12 Letter to Catherine de Fourmantel, 1.4.1760, *Letters*, 303.

13 Letter to David Garick, 31.1.1762, *Letters*, 44.

14 Letter to Mr. Foley, 14.8.1762, *Letters*, 69-71.

15 Letter to Mr. Foley, 5.10.1763, *Letters*, 86-87.

16 Letter to Mrs Fenton, *Cash, 1986*, 174.

17 Curtis LP. 'Sterne in Bond-Street', *Times Literary Supplement* 24 March 1932; 217.

18 Letter to John Hall Stevenson, 12.8.1762, *Letters*, 67

19 MacNalty A. 'Laurence Sterne: A Witty Consumptive'. *British Journal of Tuberculosis and Diseases of the Chest*, 52 (1958), 94-97.

20 Letter to the Earl of Shelburne, 1.5.1767, *Letters*, 141-142.

21 Letter (undated, and recipient unknown), 1788, *Letters*, 291.

22 Letter to Mrs James, 8.3.1768, *Letters*, 189-190.

23 *Memoirs of an Eighteenth-Century Footman*, [1790], ed. Sir E. Denison Ross and Eileen Power, 1927. 91-93. Quoted by Cash, 1986, 327.

24 St George's Hanover Square Burial Register, *1768, fol. 119*.

25 Charles Moss (1711-1802) became bishop successively of St David's and of Bath and

Wells. *Dictionary of National Biography (henceforth DNB)*. Oxford: Oxford University Press, 1988, 13: 1078-1080.

[26] This transcribes a manuscript note in Willis's copy of Sterne's Sentimental Journey. *Willis's Current Notes, 1854*. London: G. Willis, 1855, 31-32.

[27] *St James's Chronicle*, November 24-26, 1767.

[28] Clinch G. *History of Mayfair and Belgravia*. London: Truslove & Shirley, 1892, 48-56. Figure 3 from facing p. 52.

[29] Hackman H. *Wates's Book of London Churchyards*. London: Collins, 1981, 64

[30] *Public Advertiser*, March 24, 1769.

[31] Reed I. *Isaac Reed Diaries, 1762-1804*. Ed. Jones CE. Berkley and Los Angeles: University of California Press, 1946, 156.

[32] *Willis's Current Notes*. London: G. Willis, 1855, 31-32.

[33] Macalister A. *A History of the Study of Anatomy in Cambridge*. Cambridge: Cambridge University Press, 1891, 22-23.

[34] Rolleston HD. *The Cambridge Medical School*. Cambridge: Cambridge University Press, 1932, 61.

[35] Howes AB. *Yorick and the Critics*. New Haven, Connecticut: Yale University Press, 1958, 46 and n. 9; *Literary Register*. 1769, 1, 285; Cash, 332 n. 8.

[36] Sutcliff T. Woodhall and Copley Hall. *THAS* 1904-5, 251-262, and Bretton R. Woodhall, Skircoat, *THAS* 1955, 19-32.

[37] *Cash, 1986*, 353-354.

[38] Castiglioni A. *A History of Medicine*. Translated and edited by Krumbhaar EB. New York: Alfred A Knopf, 1941, 341.

[39] Langdon-Brown W. *Some Chapters in Cambridge History*. Cambridge: Cambridge University Press, 1946, 1-19.

[40] Macalister, 19.

[41] Ackermann R. *A History of the University of Cambridge*. London: R. Ackermann, 1815. Figure 14.4 is from the engraving facing p. 290.

[42] Stukeley W. *Family Memoirs of the Rev. William Stukeley, MD*. London: Surtees Society Publications, 73, 1880, 32.

[43] Masters R. *The History of the College of Corpus Christi College and the Blessed Virgin Mary ... in the University of Cambridge*. Cambridge: Cambridge University Press, 1753, 196.

[44] Charles Collignon (1725-1785). *DNB*, 1998, 4, 811-812.

[45] Macalister, 22.

[46] Collignon C. *The Miscellaneous Works of Charles Collignon, M.D.* Cambridge: F. Hodson, 1786

[47] Dainton C. *The Story of England's Hospitals*. London: Museum Press Limited, 1961.

[48] Woodward J. *To Do the Sick No Harm: A Study of the British Voluntary Hospital System to 1875*. London and Boston: Routledge & Kegan Paul, 1974.

[49] Cope Z. 'The Private Medical Schools of London (1746-1914)'. In: *The Evolution of Medical Education in Britain*. Ed. Poynter FNL. London: Pitman Medical, 1966, 89-109.

[50] Cope, Z. *William Cheselden : 1688-1752*. Edinburgh and London: Livingstone, 1953.

[51] Cooper BB. *The Life of Sir Astley Cooper, Bart*. 2 vols. London: John W Parker, 1843. Chapters 18, 19, & 20 detail Astley Cooper's extensive experience with resurrectionists.

52 Selected are: Ball JM. *The Sack-'em Up Men: An account of the rise and fall of the modern resurrectionists*. Edinburgh and London: Oliver and Boyd, 1928; Turner CH. *The Inhumanists*. London: A. Ousley Ltd, 1932; Cole H, *Things for the Surgeon*. London: Heinemann, 1964; Fido, M. *Body snatchers: A History of the Resurrectionists 1742-1832*. London: Weidenfeld and Nicolson, c.1988; Bailey B. *The Resurrection Men: a History of the Trade in Corpses*. London: Macdonald, 1991.

53 Douglas H. *Burke and Hare: the True story*. London: R. Hale, 1973.

54 Wakefield EG. *Facts relating to the Punishment of Death in the Metropolis*. London: J. Ridgway, 1831 & 1832

55 The Burkers, *Hansard*, 12.12.1831, n.s. 9, 154-155

56 Henry Warburton (1784?-1858) of Trinity College, Cambridge. *DNB*, 20, 753-754.

57 Report from the Select Committee on Anatomy, 22.7.1828. *Reports from Committees*: 7, 4, 1-150.

58 Anatomy - Subjects for dissection. *Hansard*, 12.3.1829, n.s. 20, 998-1005.

59 Withdrawal of Anatomy Bill. *Hansard*, 5.6.1829, n.s. 21, 1746-1750.

60 Schools of Anatomy. *Hansard*, 15.12.1831, 3rd.s. 9, 300-307.

61 *Cobbett's Weekly Political Register*, 28.1.1832, 75, 257-281.

62 Schools of Anatomy, 3rd reading. *Hansard*, 19.7.1832, 3rd.s. 14, 533-536.

63 *The Statutes of the United Kingdom and Ireland*. London: Eyre & Spottiswoode, 1832, 12, 891-894, 2 & 3 *Gulielmi IV*, Cap. 73-75.

64 MH74/16, *Inspector's Return*, 31.12.1842, Public Record Office, Kew.

65 Richardson, R. *Death Dissection and the Destitute*. London: Phoenix Press, 1988.

Sir Victor Horsley (1857-1916)
and the Birth of English Neurosurgery

Summary: Modern surgery developed in the second half of the nineteenth century, at the end of which neurosurgery was established as a profitable region of operative intervention.[1] In the British Isles, the first exponent was Sir William Macewen (1848-1924) in Glasgow.[2] But neuroscience had advanced in London due to the excellence of the neurologists in the several hospitals of London. The National Hospital for the Relief and Cure of the Paralysed and Epileptic, at Queen Square, opened in 1860 and provided facilities and staff in neurology.[3] Foremost among English neurosurgeons was Victor Horsley, whose career had a worldwide influence on the speciality.[3][4][5][6] Initially, operations were carried out for cranial trauma, the removal of displaced bone or blood clot, and the drainage of abscesses arising from infection of the middle ears and air sinuses. The diagnosis of brain and spinal tumours by neurologists encouraged removal by surgeons, of which Horsley was among the first.[8] Horsley performed many operations on animals, experiments opposed by the anti-vivisectionists whose campaigns Horsley countered. Horsley had many other interests, some of which displeased the establishment, and in World War I, his experience in neurosurgery was not used. He served as a general surgeon, visiting Egypt, India, and Mesopotamia where, in Amara, he died from hyperpyrexia complicating bacilliary dysentery.

Time has shown, annoyingly for his opponents, that the causes to which he devoted his life were good causes – the creation of neurological surgery, the necessity for experiments on animals, temperance if not abstinence, universal women's suffrage, the liberalism of political opinions, the need for some reforms in our profession, and Government provision of free treatment for the working man. Such variety suggests a kaleidoscopically colourful personality and makes us feel pale and desiccated beside him.[9]

Neurosurgery is considered to be one of the youngest of surgical specialties but has ancient origins that eclipse all others.[10] The oldest operation known is craniotomy which dates back to the Neolithic period, long before any written record.

The operation was trephining and skulls with trephine holes have been found throughout the world. In Europe, examples have been excavated in England, France, Denmark and Portugal. They have been found in North Africa and

148

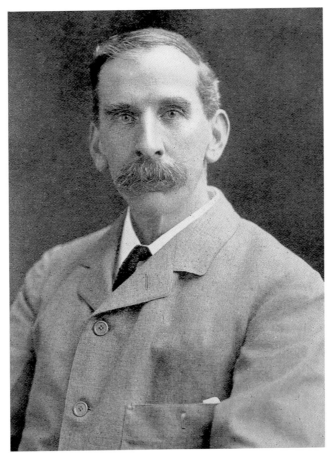

Figure 15.1. Sir Victor Horsley. Frontispiece of Paget, 1919, from which this and figures 15.3 and 15.4, are taken.

Palestine. By far the greatest number of specimens – more than ten thousand – has been discovered in the ancient mass graves of Peru. Most recovered from the craniotomy. We can only conjecture what was the purpose of these operations, so widespread in ancient times. The release of evil spirits from within the skull, for example in epilepsy, has been suggested. Interestingly, Victor Horsley wrote two papers on ancient trephining, each published in 1887, in the same year as his papers on the craniotomies he had performed.[11][12] The first surviving written account of cranial and spinal injuries (15 cases) is in the Edward Smith Surgical Papyrus,[13] written in hieratic and copied by a scribe, some three thousand years old while the text is about two thousand years earlier. Trephining was known to Hippocrates, the School of Alexandria, Roger of Salerno, Galen and Celsus. The leading surgeon of the 16th century was Ambroise Paré who performed several operations on the skull and brain. In Germany in the 17th century, both Wilhelm Fabry of Hilden and Johann Schultes (Sculteus) were prominent neurosurgeons, the latter designing many specialised instruments.

Modern neurosurgery began towards the end of the nineteenth century, being dependent on advances in surgery and the neurosciences. Surgery made great strides from two developments: anaesthesia and the control of infection. Ether anaesthesia was first used by Crawford Long (1815-1878) at Jefferson, Georgia, in 1842 and by William Morton (1819-1868) at Boston in 1846. Chloroform was first used by Sir James Young Simpson (1811-1870) in Edinburgh in 1847. Joseph Lister (1827-1912) published his first papers on antisepsis in 1867.[14] Neurology advanced more slowly but, by the end of the nineteenth century, it was developed as a specialty with attention to clinical history and physical signs. Many diseases and syndromes were identified and localisation of the disease or injury in the brain or spinal cord was achieved. Neurophysiology assisted clinical neurology. Neurosurgery was assisted by neuropathology, which identified and classified tumours of the brain and spinal cord. The stage was set for neurosurgeons. In Scotland the first was MacEwen; in England, the first was Horsley (Figure 15.1).

Horsley's Birth and Childhood

Queen Victoria gave birth to Princess Beatrice on Tuesday 14 April 1857 on which day Rosamund, the wife of John Calcott Horsley and daughter of Dr Charles Haden, produced a son at 2 Tor Villas, Campden Hill, Kensington in London. Miss Skerret, a friend of the Horsleys and a lady-in-waiting, read the announcement to the Queen who indicated that her own names be included in the names of the baby. Victor Alexander Haden Horsley was destined for greatness although in what form was unclear. His father was a painter of merit and the family included Augustus Wall Calcott, a landscape painter and Charles Edward Horsley, a musician. Dr Haden, Victor's maternal grandfather, was a physician specialising in diseases of children. Victor was a happy, bright boy, active and mischievous. He was at first left-handed but became ambidextrous. Attending Cranbrook Grammar School, he matriculated at London University in 1874. His early ambition was to be a cavalry officer but his father and a local general practitioner, Dr Thomas Joyce, directed him to medicine.

University College Medical School

Horsley entered the medical school of University College in October 1875, a vintage year as several of his fellow students later achieved distinction and were lifelong friends. Of these we may mention Francis Gotch who married Horsley's sister, Rosamund, and became professor of physiology at Oxford; Sir Fredrick Mott, a notable physician and neuropathologist; and Sir Dawson Williams, editor of the *British Medical Journal*. His teachers included: Sydney Ringer, Henry Charlton Bastian, John Russell Reynolds, Ernest Arthur Gowers and Wilson Fox in medicine, and John Marshall, Marcus Beck, Rickman James Godlee and AE Barker in surgery. John Burdon Sanderson was the professor of physiology, having

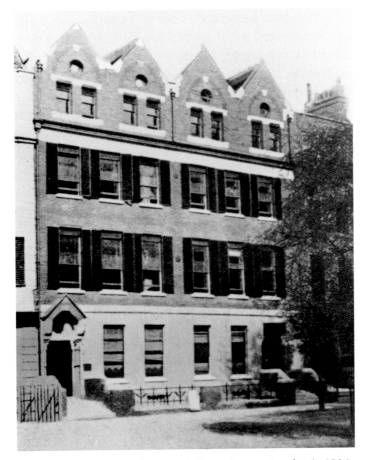

Figure 15.2 The National Hospital, Queen Square, London in 1886.

succeeded William Sharpey in the chair. Sharpey and Sanderson taught experimental physiology as the basis of medicine, which experience determined Horsley's career.[15] His enthusiasm for animal experimentation led him to a career in surgery, and to pioneer new operations in the cranial and spinal cavities. Horsley was a model student, gaining an exhibition in pathology and the gold medal in surgery. He qualified MRCS in 1880, became surgical dresser to John Marshall and clinical clerk to Henry Bastian, and obtained his MB ChB in 1881. After a post-graduate period in Germany, visiting Berlin and Leipzig, he was appointed surgical registrar at University College Hospital.

Surgical Practice, University College Hospital (UCH) and the National Hospital

In 1882 Horsley moved to 129 Gower Street from where he began private practice, at that time permitted to the UCH Surgical Registrar. He gained his FRCS in 1883 and, in 1885, was appointed Visiting Surgeon to UCH.[16] In 1886 he was elected

FRS. Edward Schafer had succeeded Burdon Sanderson at UCH and invited Horsley to assist in experiments of stimulation of the cerebral cortex, work that later was continued at the Brown Institution. Then in 1886 came an important appointment for Horsley and for neurosurgery when he became surgeon – the first – to the National Hospital, Queen Square, where he was to work for thirty years (Figure 15.2). The reputation of the physicians at the National Hospital attracted large numbers of patients who were studied expertly, and some were referred to Horsley for surgery. His facilities were poor and, at first, he operated in part of a medical ward, curtained off for the occasion. Six years later, an operating room was built but also served as a lecture room for medical students and nurses. He had no trained staff, being assisted by a house physician, sometimes with no experience of surgery, while a second house physician gave the anaesthetic. Sometimes Horsley operated alone at the house of his patient, himself administrating the anaesthetic. His excellent results, despite these primitive operating facilities, is a tribute to his operative skill, developed by performing numerous experimental operations.

In 1887 Horsley married Eldred Bramwell, after a long engagement. They lived at 80 Park Street, Grovenor Square where by now Horsley had a large private practice. They had two sons, Siward and Oswald, and a daughter, Pamela. His surgical and experimental work had brought national and international fame and in 1902 Horsley was knighted, deservedly but unexpectedly.

The Brown Institution

Thomas Brown of Dublin, who died in 1852, left £20,000 to the University of London to found the Brown Animal Sanatory Institution for research on animals useful to man. There were legal difficulties but, by the year 1871, a plot of land had been acquired, a building erected – at 146 Wandsworth Road – and the Institution opened, with John Burdon Sanderson as physician superintendent. The post provided a small salary and a house, but more important were the facilities for survival experiments on large animals – cats, dogs and primates. Sanderson was succeeded in 1878 by J Godwin Greenfield, the English neuropathologist, who then was followed by Charles Smart Roy. In 1883 Roy became Professor of Pathology in Cambridge and Horsley became the Physician Superintendent. The Superintendent chose the field of research and Horsley began a series of experiments to discover the localisation of activities of the brain, extending his work begun at University College. For this the Brown Institution was ideal, as nowhere else in London could survival experiments be performed on large animals. But Horsley enquired into diverse problems in anatomy and physiology, and into diseases of humans and animals. His experiments relating to brain function were numerous, but he also studied the thyroid and pituitary glands, and the diagnosis and control of rabies. His experiments on brain function were linked to his first

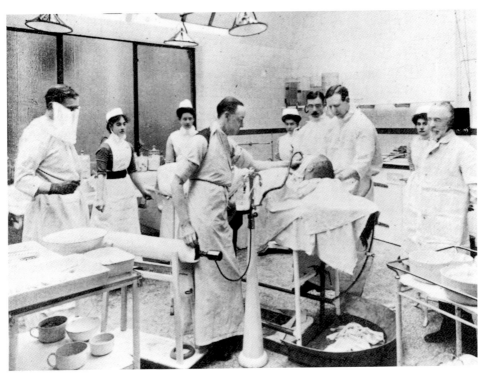

Figure 15.3 The operating theatre at Queen Square in 1906. The bearded observer on the right is Kocher, from Berne. Mr Powell is giving the anaesthetic, using the Vernon-Harcourt inhaler. Horsley, gloved and masked, is on the left. The picture was taken for use by Horsley in an address in Toronto.

operations on the brain and spinal cord, for which work he is chiefly remembered. His work on thyroid and pituitary gland function and the control of rabies will be described first.

Thyroid Deficiency

Sir William Osler (1849-1919) and others had described cretinism in childhood, and Sir William Withey Gull (1816-1890) of Guy's Hospital had distinguished the features of hypothyroidism in adults which Dr William Miller Ord (1834-1902) termed myxoedema, from the mucinoid thickening of the subcutaneous tissues.[17] Goitres were common in Switzerland and were being removed by Theodor Kocher (1841-1917) in Berne, and by the cousins Jacques and Auguste Reverdin in Geneva. These surgeons also observed that removal of the thyroid gland (or struma) gave rise to a state of weakness and asthenia to which the name *cachexia strumipriva* was given. Sir Felix Semon (1849-1921), at a meeting of the London Clinical Society on 23 November 1883, when a case of myxoedema was presented, postulated that the three conditions of cretinism, myxoedema and *cachexia strumipriva* were examples of hypofunction of the thyroid gland. On 14 December the Clinical Society formed a committee to investigate disorders of the thyroid gland, with Dr Ord as chairman. Horsley was the most active member of this committee and designed experiments on monkeys in which the thyroid gland was removed. By October 1884 these experiments had begun in Professor Schafer's laboratory at University College in collaboration with Rickman John Godlee (1849-1925). They were continued by Horsley at the Brown Institution, the experimental facilities of which were ideal. Removal of the thyroid gland in monkeys reproduced the features of myxoedema.[18] Horsley was a speedy worker and his early findings were presented in two lectures at the University of London in December 1884. The work continued in 1885 and 1886 and, in 1888, the Clinical Society published Horsley's 'Report on Myxoedema'. The findings were quickly applied to cases of myxoedema. In 1890 Horsley transplanted the thyroid gland into patients with myxoedema; in 1891 and in 1892, his pupil, George Murray (1865-1939) in Newcastle injected thyroid gland tissue, and in 1892 Hector Mackensie showed that feeding patients with thyroid gland was effective. Horsley was the prime mover of research into the thyroid, providing the experimental basis for the syndromes of thyroid deficiency and suggesting how myxoedema could be treated.[19]

The Pituitary Gland

In 1886 Horsley was the first to remove the pituitary gland in animals and his experiments were followed by others, notably Harvey Cushing in Boston.[20] Cushing described the resultant physiological state to which he gave the name *cachexia hypophyseopriva*. This comprised lethargy, drowsiness, slow respiration and lowered temperature, a syndrome that proved fatal in Cushing's experiments. Death ensued in 3-5 days in his adult dogs and in 10-30 days in his puppies. Horsley disagreed with Cushing and presented three of his experimental animals – a cat, a dog and a monkey – each of which had survived for a considerable time. In all three cases, necropsy had shown complete removal of the pituitary gland. The explanation of these conflicting reports is that Cushing – a less skilful operator than Horsley – damaged the floor of the third ventricle, which damage caused many of the adverse effects and the early deaths. Horsley was so busy with human operations and experimental work that his published accounts were less detailed than the importance of the work deserved. He had removed the pituitary gland in two animals, the first experiment of this nature.[21] In the same year, 1886, Pierre Marie (1853-1940) in Paris had described '*deux cas d' acromegalie*' although the connection of acromegaly with the pituitary gland was not appreciated before the observations of Marie and Georges Marinesco, reported in 1891. Horsley's experimental work on the pituitary gland was presented to the Physiological Society in 1911. Experiments had been performed on 54 animals (20 cats, 21 dogs, and 13 monkeys), and in 15 animals (2 cats, 9 dogs, and 4 monkeys) in which the pituitary gland was removed completely. The survivors of this group proved that complete removal of the pituitary gland does not cause death, but a syndrome of asthenia and glycosuria. Horsley also demonstrated that section of the pituitary stalk did not cause death.

Operations on Pituitary Tumours

Horsley's operations on pituitary tumours were published only briefly, regrettably as he was one of the earliest surgeons to treat acromegaly surgically. Mention of this work was made by HH Tooth (1856-1926) at the 17th International Medical Congress in London in 1913.[22] A rare monograph by G Verga, published in Pavia in 1911, reproduced Horsley's notes from his private files and the records of the National Hospital in London.[23] Ten cases are described and mention is made of two further cases. Eight survived and four died.

Rabies

Not the least of Horsley's achievements is his work on rabies, then a dangerous disease in many animals in Europe but present also in Britain. Pasteur's work on rabies in Paris and, in particular, his prophylactic treatment of subjects bitten by rabid animals, had aroused interest but also scepticism.[24] In London, the Local Government Board appointed a committee to examine Pasteur's claims, with Horsley as secretary and Sir James Paget as chairman.[25] Other members were: Sir Lauder Brunton, Dr George Fleming, Lord Lister, Sir Richard Quain, Sir Henry Roscoe and Sir John Burdon-Sanderson. Horsley, the youngest member, was the prime mover, communicating with Pasteur through the chairman and members and also arranging visits to Paris. Pasteur, overwhelmed by patients in Paris, was at first uncooperative since visitors usually expressed disbelief in his work. But Horsley impressed Pasteur who showed him his laboratory methods and gave him a rabies-infected spinal cord and two injected rabbits. Horsley returned with these and at the Brown Institution began to detect rabies by tests similar to those he had observed in Paris.[26] He also communicated Pasteur's conviction that in an island community the muzzling of all dogs and the quarantine of imported dogs would eradicate rabies. Horsley was the energetic mover in all subsequent steps to detect and eradicate rabies from Great Britain, being energetic in writing scientific reports, newspaper exhortations and in public lecturing, the last mentioned to combat the Dog Owners' Protection Association.[27] The Commission of Enquiry reported in June 1887 and the report was presented by Pasteur to the *Academie des Sciences* on 4 July. It contained the statement that Horsley's experiments, started in May 1886 'entirely confirm M. Pasteur's discovery of a method by which animals may be protected from the infection of rabies...' and went on to recommend prophylactic immunisation of persons bitten by rabid animals and the treatment of cases of hydrophobia. By 1902, the Muzzling Order and Quarantine of Imported Dogs had eradicated rabies in Great Britain. That we have been free from this contagion for over a hundred years is largely due to Horsley.

Horsley the Neurosurgeon

Horsley's neurosurgery was based on an immense experience of operations on animals. This refined his early operative technique but his animal work continued unabated throughout his career. His new experiments explored brain physiology, and the knowledge and techniques were used in the surgical treatment of human cases.

In August 1886, Horsley attended the 54th Annual Meeting of the British Medical Association at Brighton where he demonstrated three recently operated cases of Jacksonian epilepsy. Two were caused by trauma and one by a tumour. All three operations were successful in that, so far, they were free from epilepsy. The Brighton Meeting was memorable for the presence of Charcot who congratulated Horsley, not only on his operative successes but also on his many animal experiments which had helped to localise cortical function. Also present was Hughlings Jackson who commented profoundly on the three cases; his opinion was that this type of epilepsy – to which his name is now applied – could be caused by quite small lesions which should be sought and removed. It was also important to remove surrounding brain which was altered and which was the source of the epilepsy. Unfortunately Horsley, except in his Linacre Lecture, did not himself report his further work in excising cerebral cortex for epilepsy and athetosis.[28] At University College Hospital in the years 1900-1906, 30 such cases were operated upon and more operations would have been performed at Queen Square. By 1887 Horsley had performed ten brain operations and, in the following year with Gowers, he published the first case of the removal of a spinal tumour which cured the patient of paraplegia.[29] This historic case concerned a 42-year-old Army Captain whose disability began with back pain and progressed to paraplegia. After many consultations in several countries, he was seen by Dr Gowers who, diagnosing a spinal tumour, referred the case to Horsley. Horsley saw the patient at 1.00 pm on 9 June and operated that day at 3.30 pm. The operation, removing what was described as a fibro-myxoma, was a complete success and, when seen in January 1888, the patient had recovered completely. This paper of 51 pages remains a model of medical, surgical and pathology reporting, followed by a review of the literature on spinal tumours.

Sir Geoffrey Jefferson has drawn attention to Horsley's operations for trigeminal neuralgia as, during his brief career, Horsley performed more excisions of the trigeminal ganglion than any other surgeon, including Fedor Krause of Berne with whom he shared a reputation for exceptional expertise.[30] Unusually, Horsley preferred the temporal approach while his successors used the frontal route.[31] This preference arose from Horsley's extensive experience on animals which also explains his superb operative technique. He was a dextrous but gentle surgeon, with unrivalled familiarity with the structures he encountered. Horsley operated at great speed, in contrast to Cushing who, influenced by Halstead at Johns Hopkins, operated slowly.

The Horsley-Clarke stereotaxic apparatus

Robert Henry Clarke, of Cambridge and St George's Hospital, London, graduated in medicine in 1876 and became a physiologist at St George's.[32] He was the first to apply mathematical methods to neuroanatomy, thus facilitating experimental neurophysiology. Using geometrical concepts and fixed points in the cranium, he constructed an apparatus to map the brain in the cat and the rhesus monkey. First at the Brown Institute and later at University College, he collaborated with Horsley to make electrolytic lesions in the roof nuclei of the cerebellum, experiments which they published jointly.[33] This apparatus and their collaboration became famous in the history of stereotaxis in experimental physiology, which interest was revived later in the surgical treatment of a variety of cerebral disorders.[34] Clarke retired from academic physiology into general practice, having given the apparatus to FJF Barrington, a surgeon at University College. Barrington died in 1956 and the apparatus seemed lost but subsequently it was discovered in a museum of University College.[35]

Committees, National Health Insurance, Temperance and Women's Suffrage

Horsley was tireless in medical committees. He served the British Medical Association in several capacities, revived the failing Medical Defence Union by becoming its president and, for nearly ten years from 1897, was a representative on the General Medical Council. In the last mentioned body, he was one of three direct representatives chosen by the whole medical profession.[36] In these bodies he advised on death registration and the function of the coroner, on medical inspection and the treatment of school children, on state registration of nurses and on the suppression of quacks and unqualified practitioners. In these dealings, whilst he was always just with honest adversaries, his forthright manner caused much resentment. His support for a National Health Insurance scheme lost him patients and friends. His campaigns against alcohol and for the rights of women were conducted as a form of political warfare, denouncing his opponents in the press and on many platforms. His many opinions, as for example when he condemned the forcible feeding of suffragettes on hunger strike, now seem totally praiseworthy and in advance of his time.

World War I

Horsley, in the Territorial Amy for many years and with the rank of captain, was fishing in Cumberland in August 1914 when war began.[37] He returned at once to London and sought active service, but found the authorities hesitant. Such a critic of the establishment – against smoking and alcohol, and for the suffragettes – was suspect in the British Army. Both his sons enlisted in the Artists' Rifles and later were commissioned in the Gordon Highlanders. In 1915 Horsley was eventually appointed to the 21st General Hospital which in May, was to embark in *HMS Delta* for Alexandria. In the intervening weeks, impatient to serve, Horsley became Surgeon to the British Hospital established by Sir Henry and Lady Norman in the Hotel Bellevue at Wimereux near Boulogne.[38] Arriving in Alexandria, Horsley and his superiors faced the difficulties of settling the 21st General Hospital into the ancient and insanitary barracks at Ras-el-Tin. In July 1915 he was promoted to full Colonel and appointed Consultant to the Mediterranean Expeditionary Force, which increased his authority in suggesting improvements to the health of the troops and the care of the wounded. He travelled extensively, inspecting hospitals and medical units, and reporting, usually with scathing remarks, on the poor standards of care. In October he was at Anzac Cove in Gallipoli. At lunch in Alexandria an officer, recently returned from Mesopotamia, spoke of the horrors endured by the Army there and the lack of medical services which news prompted Horsley to request a transfer.[39] In March 1916 he travelled to Port Said and embarked for India where he visited Delhi and Simla, conferring with the Commander in Chief and the Director of Medical Services. In April he sailed in the hospital ship *Silicia* for Abadan and Basra. A few days later, a smaller hospital ship took him up the Tigris river to Amara. In November 1914 Basra had been taken from the Turks by British and Indian troops, who then proceeded up the Tigris and Euphrates, capturing Amara in June 1915 followed by other occupations and the taking of many prisoners. Amara, a large town situated on a narrow piece of land bounded on the West by the Tigris and to the North and East by the Mashara and Chahala canals, could only be described in terms of despair. The heat was trying at dawn, and intolerable at noon when the temperature ranged from 110-120° F in the shade. The surrounding swamps bred myriads of insects, tormenting the soldiers in their tents and bringing malaria and several other diseases. Only the prevailing wind – the Shamal – brought some relief from the stifling heat. The soldiers, when well, could scarcely bear the duties of the day. The sick and wounded were in a desperate state and their care by the medical orderlies required constant exhortation. It was here in Mesopotamia that Horsley showed the nobility of his character. His letters home describe the climate as 'hot boisterous wind and burning sun. If you get well in the wind's eye you are pleasantly cooled, because it dries you up far quicker than the sun can make you perspire, so you keep moving, therefore cooling, therefore smiling.' In work he summarised the problems confronting the medical services as 'an Augean stable'. The memorandum he despatched to the Director of Medical Services in Basra shows his concern. Sir Pardey Lukis was informed 'The Troops at the Front remain inadequately and imperfectly fed'. To the Viceroy, Lord Willingdon, he wrote 'We must have transport of all kinds' and 'All the failings of this campaign and losses due to sickness and death, are the logical outcome and inevitable result of not providing transport for the expedition'.[40] Despite his intense activity he enjoyed

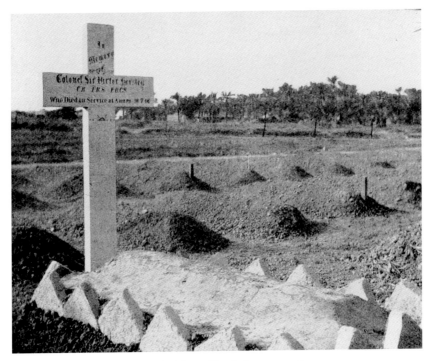

Figure 15.4 Sir Victor Horsley's grave at Amara.
The photograph was taken by Dr Andrew Balfour.

the wild life of the marshes, tracking and flushing francolins[41] and observing the edible frogs and the terrapins.

Death in Amara

On the morning of Saturday 15 July, Horsley was busy with his usual duties. He visited a RAMC captain to discuss the provision of laboratories, after which he walked back to his camp a mile and a half away. There he was informed of an officer who had become ill and he walked a further half mile to see him. By the afternoon, Horsley was complaining of headache and malaise, and was taken to hospital. Major Grey Turner spoke with him in transit but did not suspect how grave was his illness. At number 2 British General Hospital he was under the care of Major Barwell and a junior officer named Anthony Fielding, who later commented on Horsley's illness: 'He was not admitted with heat-stroke but with a mild pyrexia due in my opinion to a slight attack of Paratyphoid A, which was rampant at the time; this however was not proven bacteriologically'. On Sunday 16 July, Horsley's illness worsened, his fever progressed to hyperpyrexia, he became comatose and that evening he died. He was buried the next day in a cemetery a mile from the hospital.[42] Eighty officers attended the funeral and he was accorded full military honours. The Last Post was played and palms were strewn

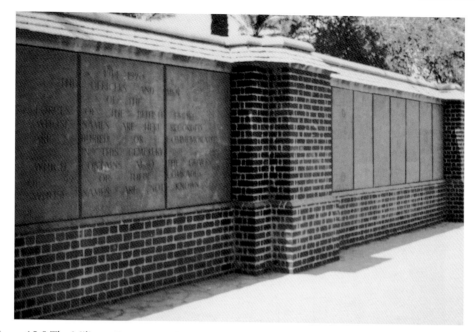

Figure 15.5 The Military Cemetery at Amara, Iraq. Recent photograph provided by the *Commonwealth War Graves Commission* to show the memorial, listing those buried in the cemetery.

over the grave, which later bore a cross of white marble (Figure 15.4). So ended tragically the life of a great surgeon, possessed of a 'kaleidoscopically colourful personality'. The Amara War Cemetery, cared for by the Commonwealth War Graves Commission, contains 4,621 burials of the First World War.[43] In 1933, all the headstones were removed and a screen wall was erected (Figure 15.5) with the engraved names of those buried in the cemetery. The War Cemetery is to the East of Amara between the left bank of the river and the Chahaila Canal.[44]

ACKNOWLEDGEMENTS

I am indebted to the Bodleian Library, in particular to its Radcliffe Science Library, for extensive facilities. David Parker of the Commonwealth War Graves Commission has kindly confirmed the recent state of the site in Amara, Irak, where Horsley was buried and has provided Figure 15.5. Access to the site is currently difficult. The biography of Paget, 1919 has been invaluable, and provided figures 15.1, 15.3, and 15.4.

NOTES AND REFERENCES

1 Balance, C,A. 'A Glimpse into the History of Surgery of the Brain. Thomas Vicary Lecture', *Lancet*, 11 (1922), 111-116 and 165-172.

2 *A History of Neurological Surgery*, edited by A Earl Walker. London: Baillière, Tindall & Cox, 1951. Horsley is described by DC O'Connor on pp. 150-151.

3 Sachs, E. *The History and Development of Neurological Surgery*. London: Cassell, 1952.

4 Bowman, A.K. *The Life and Teaching of Sir William Macewen*. London: William Hodge, 1942.

5 Holmes, G. *The National Hospital, Queen Square, 1860-1948*. London & Edinburgh: Livingstone, 1954.

6 Paget, S. *Sir Victor Horsley, A Study of His Life and Work*. London: Constable, 1919.

7 Jefferson, G. 'Sir Victor Horsley, 1857-1916'. Centenary Lecture delivered at BMA House on 12 April 1957, *British Medical Journal*, 1 (1957), 903-910.

8 MacNalty, A. 'Sir Victor Horsley: his life and work', 1957. *British Medical Journal*, 1 (1957), 910-916. Sir Arthur MacNalty had worked with Horsley at University College Hospital.

9 Lyons, J.B. *The Citizen Surgeon, A Biography of Sir Victor Horsley, FRS, FRCS, 1857-1916*. London: Peter Dawnay, 1966.

10 Mr Rickman Godlee performed the first excision of a glioma at Regents Park Hospital, now at Maida Vale. Bennett, A.H. and Godlee R.J. 'Excision of a tumour of the brain'. *Lancet*, 2 (1884), 1090-1091.

11 Jefferson, p. 910, *op cit* ref 7.

12 Thorwald, J. *Science and Secrets of Early Medicine*, translated from the German. Munich: Droemersche Verlagsanstalt, and London: Thames & Hudson, 1962.

13 Horsley, V.A.H. 'Brain surgery in the stone age'. Report of an address to the British Institution, *British Medical Journal*, 1 (1887), 582; 'Trephining in the Neolithic period', *Journal of the Anthropological Institute of Great Britain and Ireland*, 17 (1887), 100-106.

14 Horsley, V. 'Remarks on ten consecutive cases of operations on the brain and cranial cavity, to illustrate the details and safety of the method employed', *British Medical Journal*, 1 (1887), 861-866.

15 The original papyrus is in New York. It has been published by Breasted, J.H. *Edwin Smith Surgical Papyrus, in Facsimile and Hierogylphic Transliteration with Translation and Commentary*, 2 vols. Chicago: University of Chicago Oriental Institute Publications, 1930. See also: Hughes, J.T. 'The Edwin Smith Surgical Papyrus: an analysis of the first case reports of spinal cord injuries', *Paraplegia*, 26 (1988), 71-82.

16 Lister, J. 'On a new method of treating compound fracture, abscess, *etc.*, with observations on the conditions of suppuration', *Lancet*, 1 (1867), 326-329, 357-359, 507-509 and 2: 95-96.

17 Horsley subsequently published with Scharpey Schafer his work on faradic stimulation of the cerebral cortex, internal capsule, and spinal cord in primates. Horsley, V.A.H. & Sharpey-Schafer, E.A. 'A record of experiments on the functions of the cerebral cortex', *Philosophical Transactions B.*, 179 (1888-1889), 1-45.

18 Sachs, E. 'Reminiscenses of an American Student', *British Medical Journal*, 1 (1957), 916-917. Sachs, taught by Halstead at Johns Hopkins, trained with Horsley in 1907.

19 Paget, *op cit* ref 6, p. 54-67.

[20] Horsley, V.A.H. 'On the function of the thyroid gland', *Proceedings of the Royal Society of London,* 38 (1884-1885), 5-7 and 40 (1886), 6-9. Reports the experimental proof of the syndromes of thyroid deficiency.

[21] In 1905 or 1906, Theodor Kocher from Berne saw Horsley perform a thyroidectomy at UCH, and then removed a thyroid in a second patient. MacNalty, *op cit* ref 8, p. 911-912.

[22] Jefferson, *op cit* ref 7, p. 904-906.

[23] Paget, *op cit* ref 6, p. 123.

[24] Tooth, H.H. *17th International Congress of Medicine, Section XI, Neuropathology.* London: Frowde and Hodder & Stoughton, 1913, p. 161.

[25] Copies of Horsley's notes. In Jefferson, *op cit* ref 7, p. 905.

[26] On 6 July 1885, Pasteur, after many animal experiments, treated his first patient.

[27] Stephen Paget, the biographer of Horsley, was the son of Sir James Paget.

[28] Horsley also studied an outbreak of rabies in the deer in Richmond Park. Paget, *op cit,* ref 6, pp. 81-82.

[29] Horsley also examined and exposed the 'Bouisson Bath Treatment for the Prevention and Cure of Hydrophobia', Paget, *op cit* ref 6, p. 82-84.

[30] Horsley, V.A.H. 'The Linacre Lecture on the function of the so-called motor area of the brain', *British Medical Journal,* 2 (1909), 125-132. Horsley had removed the precentral area in man to treat athetosis.

[31] Gowers WR and Horsley V. 'A case of tumour of the spinal cord. Removal: recovery', *Medico-Chirurgical Transactions, London,* 53 (1888), 2nd series; 377-428.

[32] Jefferson, *op cit* ref 7, p. 906.

[33] Horsley V. 'Remarks on the various surgical procedures devised for the relief or cure of trigeminal neuralgia (*tic douloureux*)', *British Medical Journal,* 2 (1891), 1139-1143, 1191-1193, and 1249-1252.

[34] Davis, R.A. 'Victorian physician-scholar and pioneer physiologist', *Surgery, Gynecology and Obstetrics,* 119 (1964), 1333-1340.

[35] Horsley VA and Clarke, R.H. 'On the intrinsic fibres of the cerebellum, its nuclei and its efferent tracts', *Brain,* 28 (1908), 45-124.

[36] Cooper, I.S. Sir Victor Horsley: Father of Modern Neurosurgery. In *Historical Aspects of the Neurosciences,* edited by F.C. Rose and W.F. Bynum. New York: Raven Press, 1982, 235-238.

[37] Schurr, P.H. and Merrington WR. 'The Horsley-Clarke stereotaxic apparatus', *British Journal of Surgery,* 65 (1978), 33-36.

[38] Paget, *op cit* ref 6, p. 216.

[39] Lyons, *op cit* ref 9, p. 237-250.

[40] For a note on Wimereux and references see: Hughes, J.T. 'Hugh Cairns (1896-1952) and the mobile neurosurgical units of World War II', *Journal of Medical Biography,* 12 (2004), 18-24.

[41] A letter, dated 1 January 1916, states that Horsley volunteered for this transfer. Lyons, *op cit* ref 9, p. 267.

[42] Lyons, *op cit* ref 9, p. 276.

[43] Game birds.

[44] Martin Swayne described Horsley's funeral: Swayne, M. *In Mesopotamia.* London: Hodder & Stoughton, 1917.

Lawrence of Arabia and Hugh Cairns:
Crash Helmets for Motor-cyclists[1]

On a May morning in 1935, Lawrence of Arabia was fatally injured in a motor-cycle accident, which had an important sequel for thousands of future motor-cyclists. Amongst several doctors summoned to the bedside of the patient was a young brain surgeon, the first in Britain to devote himself exclusively to this specialty. Mr Hugh Cairns, Assistant Surgeon to the London Hospital, having driven a hundred miles from his home in Arundel, found the patient in a fatal coma, and was profoundly moved by the tragedy of this famous gifted young man dying, at the age of 46, inexorably from a severe head trauma. Characteristically, Hugh Cairns set about identifying, studying, and solving the problem with which he was confronted; if his recently acquired skill as a neurosurgeon could not cure or even save the life of these gravely injured patients, then perhaps the head trauma could be prevented or lessened in future. This story begins with Lawrence's accident and death in 1935 but then moves with Cairns to Oxford in 1937.

Lawrence and his motorcycle accident

Lawrence of Arabia, as he will be always known from his exploits in leading the Arab revolt against the Turks in World War I, was a man of profound mysteries fed by secretiveness and false reports, explored in many biographies.[2] If he did not actually create some of the many legends which surrounded him, at least he made no effort to diminish or dispel them. Even his true name a was a puzzle. His father was Thomas Chapman who took the name of Lawrence because he left his wife and children to live with his housekeeper, a Miss Lawrence, who, herself illegitimate, was really named Sarah Maden, and was the mother of Lawrence. This confusion of his forebears may explain why Lawrence abandoned his original name, became Ross in 1922 to enlist in the RAF as an aircraftman, but, after six weeks, joined the Royal Tank Corps in 1923 as Trooper Shaw, then returned to the RAF in 1925 as Aircraftman Shaw. His final discharge from the RAF was in February 1935.

So it was as a civilian that Mr T E Shaw, on 13th May 1935, left his cottage, Cloud's Hill, situated in Dorset near a junction on a the Dorchester to Wareham road, riding his motorcycle to Bovington Camp, a mile away (Figure 16.1). From the post office of the camp he sent a brief telegram asking Henry Williamson, the author, to come to lunch. Even this proposal later became controversial, since it seems that Williamson – a prominent supporter of the British Fascists – was not coming to discuss their common literary interests but to ask Lawrence's help at a political meeting of ex-service men at the Albert Hall, London.

163

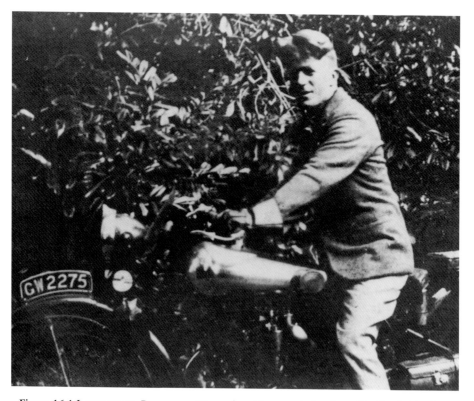

Figure 16.1 Lawrence on Boanerges. (Reproduced by permission from Yardley M. Backing into the Limelight. London; Harrap, 1985.)

Lawrence was returning to his cottage when the accident occurred. The circumstances, as revealed later at the inquest a on 21st May conducted by the Coroner, Mr L.E.N. Neville-Jones, are far from clear, mainly because of the inappropriate secrecy enjoined on witnesses by the military authorities. The secrecy was inappropriate because at the time Lawrence was a civilian, involved in an accident on a public road. There was little press coverage because the War Office requested the newspapers to publish only the statements that they issued. The Daily Sketch seems to have ignored this request (Figure 16.2). The reports concluded that he avoided an oncoming black saloon car – a mysterious vehicle never traced and seen only by one witness – and, immediately after, in overtaking two cyclists, he skidded, lost control, and pitched over the handlebars, landing in front of his machine.

Lawrence was taken in an army vehicle to the nearby hospital attached to Bovington Camp where he remained until his death in the care of the military personnel, supervised by a Captain C. P. Allen. In addition to Cairns he was visited by the neurologist, Sir Edward Farquhar Buzzard, Regius Professor of Medicine at Oxford, and the chest physician, Dr A. Hope Gosse. During the six days, during which he lay in a coma, chest complications, then inevitable in a case of prolonged

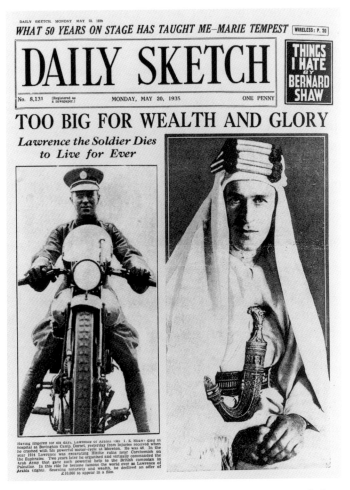

Figure 16.2 Front page of the Daily Sketch, Monday, 20 May 1935, with the notice of
Lawrence's death. (Reproduced with permission from Yardley M. Backing
into the Limelight. London; Harrap, 1985.)

unconsciousness, developed and caused his death on May 19th. The inquest –
reported in the Times on 22nd May 1935 – took place on the morning of May 21st
in a small room in the camp and the verdict was accidental death. On the same
afternoon, a large group of official mourners, including many famous names,
arrived by special train for the funeral service in the nearby Moreton church, with
burial in a small field adjacent to the graveyard.

Although this accident has been explained by the partiality of Lawrence for
speed, we find a conflict of evidence. Lawrence loved powerful motorcycles and
GW 2275 – Boanerges –, his current mount, a SS100 Brough Superior, given to him
by George Bernard Shaw and Charlotte Shaw, was sometimes described in 1935 as
the fastest motorcycle in the world. The power, acceleration and speed of this
machine outstripped its handling characteristics and braking. But people who

knew Lawrence well described him as a careful experienced rider who only indulged his liking for speed when it was safe to do so, on long straight deserted stretches of road. George Brough, the maker of the motorcycle, who had frequently driven with Lawrence described him as a very careful driver: 'I never saw him take a single risk nor put any other rider or driver to the slightest inconvenience'. So it seems wrong to assume that Lawrence's accident was due to fast reckless driving. After the accident, the gears of the cycle were found to be jammed in second gear, in which gear the maximum speed was said to be 38 mph. Lawrence was not wearing any sort of protective helmet, which then, except for motor and motorcycling racing, was not usual. From the account given above and that which follows it will be evident that a modern crash helmet remaining in position when he hit the road might have saved his life, and probably would have avoided serious permanent injury to his brain.

Hugh Cairns

The young surgeon attending Lawrence was Hugh Cairns who, born in 1896 in South Australia, qualified in medicine at the Adelaide Medical School, and, after service in World War I in the Middle East and France, came to Oxford and Balliol College as a Rhodes scholar.[3] Typically he excelled in many pursuits and in 1920 rowed bow for Oxford against Cambridge in the boat race. Cairns elected for a career in surgery and, after resident appointments in surgery in Oxford and London, in 1926-7 was sent as a Rockefeller Travelling Fellow to the United States, spending most of the time at the Peter Bent Brigham Hospital in Boston receiving a training in the new subject of neurosurgery as an assistant to Harvey Cushing. This period was study leave from the London Hospital where he had been appointed assistant surgeon with a view to developing a new department of neurosurgery. This object Cairns achieved and in 1934 became additionally honorary surgeon to the National Hospital for Nervous Diseases, at Queen Square, London. In 1935 he was the obvious choice of a neurosurgeon in the South of England to attend Lawrence.

In 1936 Cairns' future dramatically changed. The massive benefaction of Lord Nuffield to build up the medical school of Oxford included a Nuffield Chair of Surgery to which Cairns was appointed in January, 1937. His appointment was the first of several chairs and naturally Cairns had considerable influence in shaping what was virtually a new medical school. His enthusiasm and energy in building up his own department of surgery, with its new wards and offices, were remarkable and in a very short time his unit was the leading neurosurgical centre in the United Kingdom, training many of the nation's neurosurgeons and playing a very important part in the Army Medical Services in World War II (Figure 16.3).[4] His work in the Military Hospital for Head Injuries, which St. Hugh's College became from 1939-1945, has been commemorated by the installation of a plaque in the

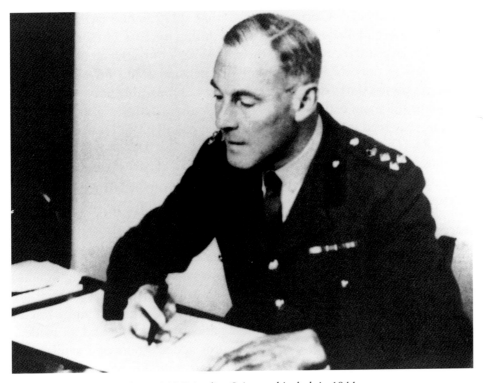

Figure 16.3 Brigadier Cairns at his desk in 1944.
(Reproduced by permission of the Oxford Department of Neurosurgery.)

College. In the 15 years following his appointment, in six of which the nation was at war, Cairns achieved a great deal, pioneering new operations and operative techniques and, importantly, initiating the first clinical trials of penicillin for Howard Florey. To meet the requirements of World War II, he devised and put into effect plans for the optimal treatment of head injuries under battle conditions. With Charles Symonds, the neurologist, he created and trained the Mobile Neurosurgical Units. These were a notable success, and some were ready before the war began in September 1939.

Wartime motorcycle accidents

During 1939 and in 1940, when occurred the swift collapse of the front in France, the evacuation from Dunkirk, and the subsequent concentration of our armed forces at home to repel invasion, battle casualties were relatively few. Some patients with head injuries, together with the No.1 Mobile Neurosurgical Unit which had accompanied the British Expeditionary Force to France, were taken prisoner. It was in this period from the beginning of the war through 1940 and including the first half of 1941, that Cairns saw so clearly the tragic and unnecessary loss of life amongst the despatch riders of the British Army. His first and most important paper on the subject appeared in the *British Medical Journal* of 4th October 1941.[5] Cairns observed that 2279 motorcyclists and pillion passengers had been killed in road accidents during the first 21 months of the war, a remarkably large total considering the relative lack of traffic on our roads in war time. Petrol was only available for military personnel and for essential civilian journeys, yet these figures were larger than for a comparable period in peace time. To determine the main cause of these deaths, Cairns analysed in detail 149 cases, discovering that head injury was the cause of death in 102 and was the only serious injury in 85. Thus head injury was by far the most important cause of death accounting, in this survey, for 68.5% of the fatalities. Non-fatal injuries in motorcyclists were much commoner, with a great range of severity, and any complete study was more difficult than an analysis of the fatalities.

Research into head injuries and crash helmets

Most significantly, however, Cairns had seen only seven cases of motorcyclists injured whilst wearing a crash helmet, and all seven were in the group of non-fatal accidents. Although the severity of the accident was sometimes as great or greater than in the fatal cases, usually with severe damage to the helmet and a fracture of the skull, the damage to the brain of these patients was slight and all made a full recovery. In the proof stage of his paper, Cairns added a note of 8 similar cases of helmeted motorcyclists surviving a severe head injury with complete recovery. Although the type of case seen by Cairns was highly selected – he did not see every mild case or those whose injury was so severe that they died before coming to a hospital –, nevertheless the evidence pointed strongly to one conclusion. In an accident, a crash helmet protected the life of a motorcyclist and reduced brain damage, even in severe trauma with a shattered helmet, to such a degree that complete recovery was the likely outcome. This first paper on this subject by Cairns attracted much attention, and editorials appeared in both the *Lancet* and the *British Medical Journal*.[6]

It was characteristic of Cairns that he not only initiated research himself, but was also a powerful stimulus to others to study the same problem with differing techniques. Already D. Denny-Brown and W. Ritchie Russell, both in the RAMC, were studying the anatomy and physiology of experimental cerebral concussion in the Oxford Physiology Laboratory, supported by the a Brain Injuries Committee of the Medical Research Council. Their extensive studies were published at length in *Brain* in a 72 page a article occupying two issues of that journal.[7] This thorough experimental work established with certainty many features of brain trauma. An important finding was that the brain within an immobilised head was much less susceptible to trauma than if the skull was allowed to move. Thus in the normal circumstance of a human accident, the movement of the head and the consequent shearing movement of the contained brain was all important.

Cairns enlisted the aid of a physicist, Dr A. H. S. Holbourn, who was attached to the Nuffield Department of Surgery and also had facilities in the Oxford

Department of Physiology.[8] Holbourn calculated the physical stresses on the human brain in an accident, and developed a theory to explain the distribution and forces operating during trauma. He also devised a model of the human brain made of 5% gelatin slightly hardened with 0.5% formalin. These models were used in a series of experiments to show the swirling effect of the brain in head trauma with rotation. The experimental findings agreed with the calculated predictions and Holbourn concluded there were two main causes of brain damage in head injuries: deformation of the skull often with fracture, and sudden rotation of the head.

By 1943 when Cairns next published on Motorcyclists, Head Injuries and Crash Helmets, with Holbourn as co-author, the data available to him had considerably expanded.[9] Since November 1941, all Army motorcyclists on duty wore crash helmets, and Cairns had now examined 106 cases of accidents in motor-cyclists wearing crash helmets. The distribution and severity of the skull fracture and brain injury was compared with the damage to the helmet. The clinical features, and particularly the period of amnesia, were related to the site of injury and type of helmet. They found that temporal blows were the most serious and occipital blows the least serious, except for injuries confined to the face when brain injury was exceptional. The study also showed a clear advantage in one type of helmet. Helmets constructed with pulp protected better than those made of vulcanised rubber.

By 1946, Cairns had gathered a large body of experience on the efficacy of the crash helmet in reducing the incidence and degree of brain injury. His paper 'Crash Helmets' was his last major publication on the subject and is packed with information then not available elsewhere.[10] With sufficient figures and time course, he was now able to show, in a graph of the monthly totals of motorcyclist fatalities (service and civilian) in Great Britain from 1939 to 1945, the decline in the numbers of fatalities that took place after November 1941, when crash helmets became compulsory wear for motorcyclists on duty. His paper concluded as follows:

> From these experiences there can be little doubt that adoption of a crash helmet as standard wear by all civilian motor-cyclists would result in considerable saving of life, working time, and the time of the hospitals.

Cairns died in 1952 from abdominal cancer, at the early age of 56, deeply mourned and with many expressions of the loss to the medical community and indeed to the whole country of such an innovative doctor. Fortunately his work on motorcyclists, crash helmets, and head injuries was carried on by the neurosurgeon, Mr Walpole Lewin.[11] We may add one more regret on the death of Cairns, that it was 21 years after he died, and 32 years after his first scientific paper on this subject, that crash helmets were made compulsory for all motorcycles riders and pillion passengers. Had Cairns lived it is unlikely that he would have allowed our legislators to be so tardy.

Development of the crash helmet

Evolutionary design of the protective helmet for vehicle users, begun by Cairns in Oxford during World War II, and originally concerned with the helmet worn by the despatch rider of the British Army, has now expanded into research on all types of helmets for civilian and military personnel. Helmets are now common, not only for vehicular transport, but also for dangerous work (the hard hat), and many sports. Several countries have greatly expanded research on protective helmets and introduced legislation compelling the use of helmets. In the United Ringdom, the British Standards Institution produced the first specification (BS1869) for Crash Helmets in 1952, and subsequently have issued many relevant specifications on this subject, not only concerning protective helmets for motorcyclists, but also for racing motorcyclists and racing motor car drivers. The methods of testing helmets have also been regulated by PD 6476 issued by the BSI in 1976. A standard for protective helmets for motorcyclists (BS6658) was issued by the BS1 in 1985 and was reviewed by Glaister of the RAF Institute of Aviation Medicine, Farnborough.[12]

The voluminous literature on road and other accidents and particularly that of motorcycle accidents, described as a 'modern epidemic' [13] [14] [15] emphasises the current concern with prevention. It has been interesting to trace back this research to Hugh Cairns in Oxford in World War II, and then further still to May 13th 1935, when a motorcycle accident caused the death six days later of Lawrence of Arabia, a famous hero of World War I.

REFERENCES

[1] The British Association for the Advancement of Science met in Oxford in September, 1988. This article is based on the exhibit on Lawrence and Cairns, which was part of the exhibition 'The Growth of a County Hospital, 1920-1988.

[2] Williamson, H. *Genius of Friendship, T E Lawrence*. London: Faber and Faber, 1941; Weintraub, S. *Private Shaw and Public Shaw, a dual portrait of Lawrence of Arabia and G.B.S.* London: Jonathan Cape, 1963; Brent P. *T E Lawrence*. London: Book Club Associates, 1975 ; Stewart, D. *T E Lawrence*. London: Hamish Hamilton, 1977; Yardley, M. *Backing into the Limelight, a Biography of T E Lawrence*. London: Harrap, 1985.

[3] Obituaries: Lancet, 26th July, 2 (1952), 202-203 and *British Medical Journal*, 26th July, 2 (1952), 233-234.

[4] Cope, Z. Chapter 10, 'Neurosurgery', in *Surgery: History of II World War*. London: HMSO, 1953.

[5] Cairns, H. 'Head Injuries in Motor-cyclists, the importance of the crash helmet', *British Medical Journal*, 2 (1941), 465-483.

[6] Editorials: 'Head Injuries in Motor-cyclists', *British Medical Journal*, 2 (1941), 481 and 'Head Injuries', *Lancet*, 2 (1941), 801-802.

[7] Denny-Brown, D and Russell, W.R. 'Experimental Cerebral Concussion', *Brain*, 64 (1941), 93-164.

[8] Holbourn, A.H.S. 'Mechanics of Head Injuries', *Lancet*, 2 (1943), 438-441.

[9] Cairns, H and Holbourn A.H.S. 'Head Injuries in Motor-cyclists, with special reference to crash helmets', *British Medical Journal*, 1 (1943), 592-598.

[10] Cairns, H. 'Crash Helmets', *British Medical Journal*, 2 (1946), 322-4.

[11] Lewin, W and Kennedy W.F.C. 'Motor-cyclists, crash helmets, and head injuries', *British Medical Journal*, 1 (1956), 1253-1259.

[12] Glaister, D.H. 'Protective helmets for motor-cyclists – a new British Standard' (BS6658), *Injury*, 17 (1986), 376-379.

[13] Gissane, W. 'A study of 183 road deaths in and around Birmingham in 1960'. *British Medical Journal*, 2 (1961), 1716-1720.

[14] Bothwell, P.W. 'The problem of motor-cycle accidents', *Practitioner*, 182 (1962), 474-488.

[15] Avery, J.G. 'Motor-cycle accidents in teenage males, a modern epidemic', *Practitioner*, 222 (1979), 369-380.

Hugh Cairns (1896-1952) and the
Mobile Neuro-Surgical Units of World War II

Summary In World War II, Hugh Cairns, Oxford Nuffield Professor of Surgery, and Brigadier in the *Royal Army Medical Corps*, designed, and administered the *Mobile Neuro-Surgical Units* which treated casualties with head injuries in the various campaigns fought by the British Army. Cairns also created the *Combined Services Hospital For Head Injuries at St Hugh's College, Oxford*, where the staff of the Units were trained, and where evacuated casualties were received. The excellent outcome of the head-injured in World War II, and the impetus to the expansion of neurosurgery in the United Kingdom during and after World War II was, in large measure, due to Cairns. Others had knowledge of neurosurgery, but Cairns inspired surgeons, neurologists, and nursing sisters to perform neurosurgery, at the highest level, on the battlefield.

In the wards of the neurosurgical unit, British soldiers lay side by side with Indians, Ghurkas, Jugoslavs, Albanians, and German wounded prisoners-of-war. ...Their common bond was a bullet in the brain and the necessary operations to extract it.[1]

In World War I, head injuries from the trench warfare in Belgium and France were treated by surgeons of the Royal Army Medical Corps (RAMC), not previously trained in neurosurgery, an exception being Percy Sargent of London. The Americans made a notable contribution under the direction of Harvey Cushing.[2] There was some segregation of head wounds – e.g. at Etaples and Wimereux – and surgeons, such as G. Jefferson, W. W. Wagstaffe and R. Whitaker, began neurosurgery in the war, and did creditable work.[3] The prognosis of a penetrating wound into the brain was grave, and many patients died, mainly from secondary infection. Without antibiotics, prevention of infection was difficult and treatment almost impossible. Sir Almoth Wright stated the problem succinctly: instruments could be sterilised with antiseptics, but antiseptics would not sterilise wounds.

In World War II (WWII), outcome improved: most head-injured patients recovered, and many returned to their units for active service. The four important developments were: expert neurosurgery in the battlefield; anti-bacterial therapy, notably penicillin; speed of evacuation, especially by air; and the specialism of the *Combined Services Hospital for Head Injuries at St Hugh's College, Oxford*. Hugh Cairns figured in all of these developments, but this article focuses on the *Mobile Neuro-Surgical Units* (MNSUs) of the RAMC. These were conceived, planned, formed, trained, and directed by Cairns.

Life of Cairns

Hugh William Bell Cairns[4] was born in South Australia, and qualified in medicine at Adelaide Medical School, his medical studies being interrupted by World War I. He enlisted as a private in the Australian Army Medical Corps, but, contracting typhoid fever, was sent home to finish his medical studies, rejoining his Corps as a Regimental Medical Officer in France, and serving to the end of the war. A Rhodes Scholarship brought him to Oxford in 1919 to study anatomy and physiology. Resident posts at the Radcliffe Infirmary, Oxford, were followed by others at the London Hospital, Whitechapel, where, in 1926, he was appointed to the Surgical Honorary Staff. Later that year he was awarded a Rockefeller Travelling Scholarship for a year to train in neurosurgery with Harvey Cushing at the Peter Bent Brigham Hospital, Boston. He returned to the London Hospital, becoming a full surgeon in 1933, but his plans for a neurosurgical unit at the London Hospital altered when in 1937, he was appointed as the first Nuffield Professor of Surgery at Oxford. By the spring of 1938, he had moved to Oxford and was building his department of neurosurgery, bringing several staff from London, notably Joe Pennybacker. War with Germany was expected and Cairns began planning the MNSUs for the battlefields, and a hospital for head injuries in Oxford – *The Combined Services Hospital for Head Injuries, St Hugh's College* – , in which, neurosurgeons, neurologists, anaesthetists, theatre sisters, and ward sisters were trained in handling head injuries, of the type and numbers expected in battle.[5][6] His other notable achievement in wartime was to introduce crash helmets for army despatch riders, substantially reducing the mortality and morbidity of their road accidents.[7]

The Mobile Neuro-Surgical Units

A MNSU consisted of a neurosurgeon, a neurologist, an anaesthetist, two general duty medical officers, two nursing sisters trained in managing neurosurgical cases, and four RAMC other ranks. Two drivers of the Royal Army Service Corps maintained and drove the vehicles (Figure 17.1), which carried all equipment required for neurosurgery. A petrol engine and generator provided power for theatre lighting, heating of the two operating tables, surgical diathermy, a motor pump for suction, and sterilisation of theatre bowls and instruments (Figure 17.2). Two large pressure paraffin stoves were also used for sterilisation. The MNSU was attached to a Casualty Clearing Station (CCS) or to a Base Hospital, where the patients were housed, nursed, and fed. Local RAMC and nursing staff were added, enabling the MNSU to mount three teams, dealing continuously with several hundred casualties, for which sufficient materials were carried. There were nine MNSUs but the first (not numbered) was captured in France in 1940, and MNSUs 7 and 8 were assembled for the war with Japan, despatched to India, but, Japan

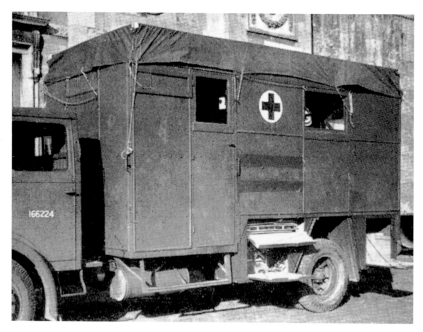

Figure 17.1 Ambulance truck of the first MNSU, in 1940 outside the Nuffield Institute of Medical Research, now Green College, Oxford.

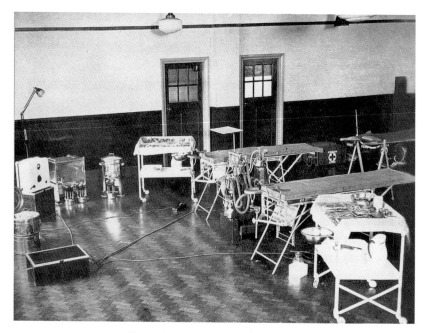

Figure 17.2 Equipment of a MNSU.

having surrendered, did not treat new battle casualties. Thus we are concerned with six MNSUs, nos. 1-6, whose work was summarised, after the war, by Cairns.[8]

The official account of the RAMC in World War II was recorded by a group of experts, dealing with different campaigns, under the direction of F.A.E. Crew.[9] The MNSUs shadowed the major campaigns fought by the British Army in WW II. They also dealt with most of the head injuries in the Royal Navy and the Royal Air Force. The Royal Navy created a *Naval Neurosurgical Unit*, first at Plymouth, then, after bombing of that city, at Sherborne.[10] Other allied forces performed neurosurgery on casualties. In North Africa, the Australians – *The Australian Imperial Force* – formed a Neurosurgical Unit which saw much service.[11] In Italy, the Canadians – *The Royal Canadian Army Medical Corps* – formed a Mobile Neurosurgical Unit attached to 21 Army Group.[12] *The Canadian Neurological Hospital at Basingstoke* also had a neurosurgical unit.[13] These separate units and hospitals were closely integrated, with uniform care to civilians and members of the armed forces of any nation. The American experience of neurosurgery in WW II was immense, but is outside the scope of this account.

France in 1940

The first MNSU, commanded by Major W.R. Henderson, arrived in France in 1940. A few days later, in the night of May 9-10, the Bock and Rundstedt Army Groups invaded Belgium, Holland, and Luxembourg, beginning their swift breakthrough into France. The MNSU, attached to a Casualty Clearing Station, overwhelmed by the enemy, found itself in charge of 800 general casualties. The nursing staff had been evacuated, but Major Henderson and his other staff passed into captivity, and spent the remainder of the war in prisoner-of-war camps, practising such surgery as was possible. Two lessons were learnt: that such a highly trained unit should not risk capture lightly and that, when military disaster ensues, little specialised surgery is possible.

North Africa, Sicily, and Italy

MNSU no.1 was formed in the winter of 1942, and consisted of Major P.B. Ascroft, neurosurgeon;[14] Major M. Kremer, neurologist; Major R.W. Cope, anaesthetist; and Major R.S. Hooper and Captain G.B. Northcroft, assistant surgeons. The Unit proceeded to North Africa, joining the Eighth Army in the Western Dessert. Their first tour of duty was from November 1941 to February 1942, during which many lessons were learnt in performing surgery in a swiftly moving theatre of war. Rapid advances were followed by swift withdrawals as the lines of battle were adjusted. MNSU no.1 covered some 2,500 miles, worked in 24 locations, admitted 336 patients, and performed 238 operations. However, only 27 cases were neurosurgical – another lesson: it was difficult to concentrate specialised cases in a fluid campaign. The Unit learnt how to open in a new

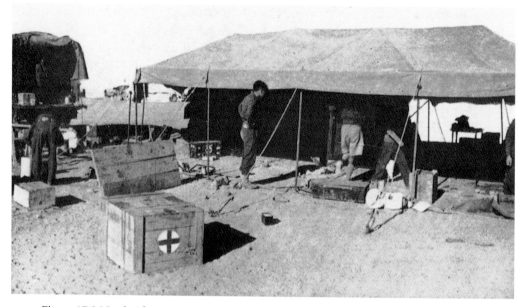

Figure 17.3 North Africa. Erecting a Neurosurgical Operating Theatre in the Eighth Army.

location with great rapidity (Figure 17.3), and also, how to pack up and move. When Rommel attacked Benghazi in January 1942, the Unit was within an hour of capture, but withdrew safely, with all vehicles, staff and equipment. The Unit resumed work in Cairo, attached to the 15th Scottish Hospital, where much neurosurgery was performed.

On the night of October 23, 1942, the battle of El Alamein began, with large numbers of casualties – 13,500 men in twelve days.[15] The battle had similarities to that of the Somme in World War I, as the defensive position was held on both sides by massive forces of infantry, armour, and artillery and, situated between the Mediterranean and the Qattara Depression, could not be outflanked. The numerous casualties had rapid expert treatment and swift evacuation, in which MNSU no.1, soon to be joined by MNSU no.4, played a vital role.

MNSU no.4, consisted of Major K. Eden, neurosurgeon;[16] Captain S.H. Llewellyn-Smith, neurologist; Major R.P. Harbord, anaesthetist; Captain H.S. Slemon, surgeon; and Captain F.J. Gillingham, general duties officer. The Unit joined the Eighth Army in Cairo in December 1942 and, after the breakthrough, went forward with the Eighth Army across Cyrenaica into Tripolitania and Tunis. This Unit used a flexible strategy suitable to the long lines of evacuation, with a forward section near the front line and a rear section, at Tripoli, from where an air service evacuated cases to MNSU no.1 at Cairo. Kenneth Eden pioneered forward mobile neurosurgery, using a 10-ton diesel motor-coach captured from the Italians and fitted out as an operating theatre, with a central table, and trays for instruments and dressings fixed to the walls. Lighting came from batteries,

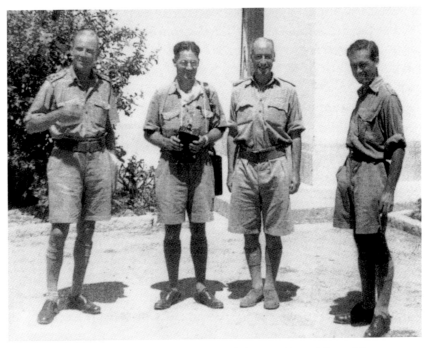

Figure 17.4 Penicillin trials in the Eighth Army. From left to right:
Brigadier H.B. Cairns, Howard Florey, Lt. Col. J.S. Jefferey, Major P.B. Ascroft.

recharged by running the engine, and a headlight came from an electrical point in the ceiling. At the back was a 'scrubbing up' facility, more stores, and a table for writing notes. An adjacent tent, connected by a canvas corridor, was a pre-operation ward, which could accommodate a dozen casualties awaiting surgery. This self-contained operating theatre could arrive and begin work within an hour and, equally important, could depart as speedily. Results were excellent as Cairns wrote:

> he [Eden] was able to excise and close the majority of the head wounds of the Eighth Army within 24 hours, and to obtain over 90% of primary healing, a great improvement on anything previously seen in this war, for on all fronts up to date the incidence of brain abscess after brain wounds has been high.

The overall organisation of surgery in the RAMC in Africa was described by Major General Ogilvie.[17] Most unfortunately Eden was to die from poliomyelitis.[18] MNSU no.4, now under the command of Major F.J. Gillingham,[19] proceeded to Sicily, where the Allies had parachuted on 9 July, and landed on 10 July, 1943. Rapid military success – in thirty eight days – limited casualties, on which MNSUs nos.4 & 5 made the first trials of penicillin in neurosurgery.[20] Mussolini abdicated on 25 July, but the Germans, who had not defended Sicily, moved many troops into Italy. On 3 September, the Eighth Army invaded Italy, landing near Reggio from nearby Sicily, whilst, on 5 September, the US Fifth Army landed on Salerno,

South of Naples. German opposition was fierce and, moving North, the Allies were halted at the formidable Gothic Line – from Rimini to Pisa.

MNSU no.4 divided in two for the *Battle of the Gothic line*, the forward section being at Loretto, whilst the rear section was 400 miles South, at Barletta. Fighting was fierce and, in 54 days, 987 neurosurgical casualties were admitted, overwhelming the resources of the forward section, in which, at one time, there were 52 cases awaiting operation. Subsequently the *Battle of the Po valley* had even greater casualties, but the Unit, with reinforced personnel, coped. One feature at the rear section of MNSU no.4 at Barletta was the arrival of untreated Jugoslav head injuries from the Balkans, demonstrating the horrific consequences of delayed treatment of head wounds.[21] Connolly wrote: 'Many of the patients had had long and difficult journeys fron the interior of Yugoslavia, often receiving only the bare minimum of medical attention.' There were 113 cases of unhealed brain wounds, complicated by brain abscesses, meningitis and ventricultis, and a varied flora of pathogenic organisms. There were 23 deaths, not a great mortality in such neglected cases, for which penicillin was not available. During its existence, MNSU no.4 admitted 6063 cases on which 4334 operations were performed, almost all on head injuries.

MNSU no.5, was commanded by Major J. Schorstein[22] and formed in the Autumn of 1942. Schorstein was trained in Manchester, as were Captains R.P. Jepson and K. Tutton, who, at Schorstein's request, were posted to this Unit, which became known, unofficially, as the Manchester MNSU, and was joined by Captain C.W.M. Whitty, neurologist. The Unit left England in December 1942 with the First Army, landing in North Africa as part of *Operation Torch* and, in the subsequent weeks, received many casualties in a campaign with a wide front, difficult lines of communication, and air evacuation less developed than in the Eight Army. With the total success of the First and Eighth Armies in North Africa, MNSU no.5 proceeded briefly to Sicilly, and then to Italy. In Italy, MNSU no.5 divided into a forward section near the battle, and a rear section near an airfield for evacuation. The *Battle of Monte Cassino* was memorable for the number of casualties: Captain Whitty in the rear section, attached to 65 General Hospital at Naples, admitted 333 cases of head injuries between May 12 and May 26. During its existence, MNSU no.5 admitted 4600 casualties and performed 2239 operations. The campaign in Italy ended on 28 April, when the German forces surrendered to General Alexander.

Europe after D-day

MNSU no.6, commanded by Major J.M. Small[23], neurosurgeon, with Captain E.A. Turner and Major A.C. Watt, joined the 21st Army Group in France soon after the Normandy landings of *Operation Overlord* on 6 June 1944, when 156,000 men were put ashore. The breakout from the invasion beaches was achieved,

Montgomery launched his offensive on 18 July, and the Americans, further West, broke through on 25 July. The German counter offensive failed and the landing, mostly of American troops, in the South of France on 15 August enabled a broad sweep of the Allies through France. Paris was liberated on 26 August, and the bridges across the Rhine – except for Arnheim – were secured by 17 September. The offensive lost momentum until the spring when, in March, 1945, the Rhine was crossed in force, and Germany was invaded. Overwhelming ground forces and total air superiority in the West matched the success of the Russian Armies in the East. On 30 April, Hitler committed suicide and, on 7 May, the Germans surrendered unconditionally.

In a campaign of less than one year, MNSU no.6 moved with the invading armies, being attached either to a CCS or to a Base Hospital, and sometimes split into forward and rear sections. There were notable differences from the earlier campaigns. Accommodation was rarely less than a well equipped tented hospital, more often was in suitable buildings, and, in Brussels, within a modern hospital. Treatment of cases was near ideal. The general surgeons in the Field Ambulances and CCSs were able to sort head injuries, passing to the MNSU those that penetrated the dura into the brain. They retained and operated on those with scalp wounds and skull fractures with intact dura, allowing the Unit to concentrate on the most grave cases. Another favourable feature was rapid air evacuation either to a base hospital or to St Hugh's, Oxford, sometimes on the same day of their injury. By June 1945, the Unit had admitted 3100 casualties, of which 1110 were penetrating wounds.

The Eastern Theatre

We now turn to Eastern Bengal, Assam, and Burma, where the conditions experienced by MNSUs no.2 and 3 could scarcely be more different than those in North West Europe. That operating standards were maintained under the most exacting conditions merits high praise.

The Japanese attacked Pearl Harbour on 7 December, 1942, but, on the same day, their troops landed in Eastern Malaya. Having overrun Malaya and taken Singapore, they were poised to invade Burma, and thence India. Rangoon was in Japanese hands, removing the only effective port from which the Allies could supply a campaign which involved Burma and Assam.

The central position was Imphal some fifty miles East of the Chindwin river, and the junction of two mountain roads running south to Tamu in the East and Tiddim in the West and a road running north 130 miles to Dimapur. These 'roads' were improved mule or bullock tracks. At Dimapur a single line railway of one metre gauge reached the Bramaputra river, which was crossed by ferry – there was no bridge. Another small gauge railway led to a broad-gauge railway with some hundreds of miles to Calcutta. These precarious lines of communication were used for all supplies from India to the thousands of troops fighting on a front of hundreds of miles in the mountainous border between Assam and Burma. The sick and wounded had to be evacuated along the same route, and this was the easy part of their journey. To reach expert surgery from the battle often required great distances, either walking, carried by stretcher, or moved by primitive boats. To this mountain terrain were added many difficulties. The heat and humidity were intense, and all accounts mention lassitude from minor illnesses, and incomplete recovery from major diseases, such as dysentery (amoebic and bacillary), cholera, scrub typhus, malaria, and hepatitis. Richard Johnson[24] described a medical officer who:

> at the end of a weary day's march, sat up all night by the banks of a stream and injected the water, doctored with a little salt, into the veins of a patient with cholera, so saving his life, and it all had to be done with a 10c.c. syringe.

Smallpox was rife in the native population. Food was often insufficient and unpalatable. Supplies of drugs, instruments, and dressings were often inadequate and many substitutes were contrived.

MNSU no.2, commanded by Major B.B. Hickey, joined the 14th Army, first in Poona, then Bangalore. The Unit moved into the battle area at Dimapore, described above, and operated under arduous conditions from March 1952 to June 1945. Details of their work are sparse but, during 1944, 443 operations were performed on head injuries.[25]

MNSU no.3, commanded by Major R. Johnson,[26] landed in India, and worked in Ranchi, Bareilly, Imphal, and other places on the mobile battle lines. At Imphal, the forward Unit was attached briefly to an Indian General Hospital, but a dugout covered by a tent was the more usual operating theatre. By early 1944, Imphal was being supplied by air, enabling air evacuation of casualties on the return flights to the rear section at Comilla, in Eastern Bengal. A C47 (Dakota) could transport 18 lying and 5 sitting casualties. Smaller aircraft were also used, for example, the LS (Stinson Reliant), a high wing monoplane that accommodated one casualty.

At Comilla, a substantial Head Injury Centre was created – supplied mostly by air – and much neurosurgery performed. But Comilla, in the plains of East Bengal was most unhealthy – the heat and humidity was intense, there was no air conditioning, and it was preferable to perform operations at night. Procedures differed from those anticipated in a 1941 booklet to Junior Medical Officers in India:

> There is no reason why you should not visit your patients at other times than the official round. It is a good policy occasionally to walk round your ward in the afternoon or evening, even when you may not be on orderly duty.

And on recommending rounds on a horse:

> You will see more from the back of a horse than you will from a car, a bicycle or on foot – 'The sweetest wind from heaven is that which bloweth between the ears of a horse.'– Persian proverb[27]

Cairns sent his RAMC surgeons into India and Burma with more urgent instructions. The most seriously wounded – perhaps the lucky ones – were evacuated after primary surgery at Imphal by air to Comilla, from which the British troops were transferred to military hospitals at Bangalore and Secunderabad. Less seriously wounded went by the route mentioned above, of which Johnson wrote:[28]

> jeeps were used …with three stretcher racks and although the method had the advantage of speed where the track was good enough, there was no shelter from the sun or rain and the dust which formed a cloud which never settled and crept into everything. It found a ready entrance to the nose, ear, hair and clothes and was laden with organisms including the Bacterium Coli. …The driver wore goggles and a wet handkerchief over the mouth and nose.

This was the evacuation after primary surgery, before which, after wounding, the journey over mountainous terrain, on foot, by stretcher, on mule, or carried by a single porter, varied, but was always a feat of endurance. An example was a sergeant with a bullet in his frontal lobe, which had entered through the optic foramen and destroyed his eye. With his wound covered by a simple field dressing, he walked 90 miles to the MNSU where, after operation, he was evacuated. That he made a good recovery, emphasises what can be done under such adverse conditions.

To their great credit, the British Army, whose United Kingdom Units were supported by Indian, West African, Asian, and Dominion troops, overcame the difficulties of the Burma Campaign. The Japanese initially held the rivers, railways, and roads, and the port of Rangoon. Air supply was the key to the allied military success and groups, which became surrounded, were massively reinforced by air. The tide turned and the Battle of Imphal - not well known at home – was as important in the Far East as that of El Alamein was in North Africa.

MNSU no.3, in total, admitted 2045 casualties, operated on 1200, of which 1100 were head injuries. Peripheral nerve injuries were also treated, and assistance was given to MNSU no 2 by taking 235 of their Burma casualties in 1945.

The Treatment of Head Injuries

Handling of head-injured casualties was greatly refined during WW II; modifications were introduced as lessons were learnt. The basic intracranial operation was exploration of the wound by a nearby burr-hole, removal of dead tissue, bone fragments, blood clot, and foreign material, including metallic bodies if easily accessed, and, if possible, primary closure of the dura and scalp. Suction and good lighting of the operation was essential and available in every MNSU. The interval between injury and neurosurgery varied greatly, but primary operation by the staff of a MNSU was preferable to early surgery by surgeons inexperienced in head wounds.

What has been described refers to wounds of the vertex, but wounds to the face, eyes, and ears were now treated by maxillo-facial units, and ophthalmic, ENT, dental, and plastic surgeons assisting the MNSUs. Casualties with multiple injuries, for example, major injuries to the spine, chest or abdomen, were also treated by a combination of surgeons. Longer term was the reconstruction of the cranium by what might be termed 'plastic neurosurgery'.

After the Battle of *El Alamein*, results improved substantially: when the campaign was going well, medical treatment could be well organised and maximally effective. A large scale trial of penicillin in 5 hospitals at Tripoli and Sousse in 1943 demonstrated its efficacy in combating infections (Figure 17.4). In the Battle of Sicily, in July and August, 1943, MNSUs 4 & 5 used penicillin locally in head wounds, with obvious benefit, and subsequently in Italy, with many more cases, the value of penicillin in combating infection proved outstanding.[29] [30] The MNSUs rapidly developed a regime of local and systemic antibiotics which became standard treatment.

Evacuation, by air and eventually to the UK, was greatly developed by the RAF, and experienced staff accompanied the casualties. Selection of cases, usually by the neurologists, was critical. Restless patients travelled well, provided morphia was withheld, but comatose patients required turning to avoid chest complications. Above all, the first neurosurgical operation must have been correctly performed. Finally, all medical and nursing staff in contact with the MNSUs became aware of the special needs of head injuries, and how much recovery was possible with expert treatment, as Cairns wrote:[31]

> even the experienced nurse might have found a ward full of patients with head wounds an almost insupportable sight, including as it did many who were in deep coma, others violently or vocally restless, and yet others, who, though docile, were irresponsible. Some required intravenous drip or tube feeding, some had to be restrained.

Nursing Sisters arriving from St Hugh's Hospital, well versed in attending neurosurgical cases, were always welcomed into the Military Hospitals, bringing a skill valued by Principal Matrons.

Post World War II

War frequently brings medical advances, and WW II caused expansion of neurosurgery in the United Kingdom. Additional to the work of Cairns in Oxford, was that of Geoffrey Jefferson, based in Manchester, but overseeing neurosurgery in several of the *Emergency Medical Hospitals* throughout the United Kingdom.[32] Other neurosurgeons busy with head injuries were Dott in Edinburgh and Rowbotham[33] in Newcastle. Then, in 1948, the creation of the National Health Service allowed expansion of existing neurosurgical centres, and creation of others. To these old and new neurosurgical departments came the surgeons, whose army career we have followed. In London, Sir Charles Symonds was active in founding the Guy's-Maudsley Neurosurgical Unit, with Murray Falconer as its first director. Ascroft returned to the Middlesex Hospital, and Johnson, Schorstein, and Jepson to Manchester, where Johnson was to succeed Jefferson in the chair of Neurosurgery. Gillingham, Lewin, and Tutton became Professors of Neurosurgery at Edinburgh, Cambridge, and Preston, and Small became the senior neurosurgeon at Birmingham.

Neurosurgery at Oxford suffered a reverse on the death of Cairns from abdominal cancer in 1952 at the early age of 56. His chair was of Surgery, and, when filled by a thoracic surgeon, the impetus to neurosurgery was lost. But Cairns's successor, Joe Pennybacker, was revealed as the outstanding diagnostician and operative surgeon, whose work had underpinned that of Cairns, and who, at Oxford, trained several generations of neurosurgeons, from many countries.

ACKNOWLEDGEMENTS

I am indebted to the Bodleian Library, in particular to its Radcliffe Science Library, for extensive facilities. I thank the Wellcome Trust for the use of papers in the RAMC Muniment Collection of the Wellcome Library for the History and Understanding of Medicine.

NOTES AND REFERENCES

[1] Peripatetic Correspondent. *Lancet* 1944; ii: 832.

[2] Cushing, H. *British Journal of Surgery*, 5 (1917-1918), 558-684.

[3] Jefferson G. 'Head Wounds and Infections in Two Wars', *British Journal of Surgery, War Supplement no. 1*, 1947 (henceforth *BJSWS*), 3-8. The % mortality of wounds penetrating the dura was: Cushing 41.4% ; Jefferson 36.7 ; Wagstaffe 50% ; and Whittaker 9.3%. Whittaker's cases may have been selected.

[4] Fraenkel, G.J. *Hugh Cairns*. Oxford: Oxford University Press, 1991.

[5] Schurr PH. The Contribution to Neurosurgery of the Combined Services Hospital for Head Injuries at St Hugh's College, Oxford, 1940-1945, *Journal of Royal Army Medical Corps*, 134 (1988), 146-148.

[6] Cairns ruled St Hugh's, but nominally in charge were Air Vice-Marshall C.P. Symonds, Consultant in Neuropsychiatry to the Royal Air Force, and Brigadier G. Riddoch, Consultant Neurologist to the British Army.

[7] Hughes, J.T. Lawrence of Arabia and Hugh Cairns: crash helmets for motorcyclists, *Journal of Medical Biography*, 9 (2001), 236-240.

[8] Cairns, H. 'The Organization for Treatment of Head Wounds in the British Army'. *British Medical Bulletin*, 3 (1945), 9-14; and Neurosurgery in the British Army, 1939-1945. *BJSWS*, 9-26.

[9] The RAMC in WW II is described in Crew, F.A.E. *The Army Medical Services. Campaigns*: Vol. 2. Includes Libya and North-West Africa 1942-1943; Vol. 3. Sicily, Italy,

and Greece, 1944-1945; Vol. 4. North-West Europe 1944-1945; and Vol. 5. Burma. London: HMSO, 1957, 1959, 1962, and 1966.

[10] Rogers, L. 'Neurosurgery in the Royal Navy', *BJSWS* 90-95.

[11] Miller, D. 'Infective Complications of Head Battle Casualties', *Australian and New Zealand Journal of Surgery,* 12 (1942-1943), 55-63.

[12] Slemon, H.V. 'Forward Neurosurgery in Italy', *Journal of Neurosurgery,* 2 (1945), 332-339.

[13] 'The Canadian Neurosurgical Centre, Hackwood Park, Basingstoke', *British Journal of Surgery,* 32 (1944-1945), 525-530.

[14] Ascroft, P.B. 'Treatment of Head Wounds due to Missiles', *Lancet,* 1943; 2: 211-218. Ascroft's papers dealing with MNSU no. 1 are in the *RAMC Muniment Collection, Wellcome Library for the History and Understanding of Medicine,* 1154, boxes 257 & 258.

[15] Churchill, W.S. *The Second World War,* volume 4. London: Cassell, 1951, 541.

[16] Eden, K. 'Mobile neurosurgery in warfare', *Lancet,* 2 (1943), 689-692.

[17] Ogilvie, W.H. 'War Surgery in Africa', *British Journal of Surgery,* 31 (1943-1944), 313-324.

[18] Obituary, 'Kenneth Eden', *Lancet,* 2 (1943), 653.

[19] Gillingham, F.J. 'Neurosurgical Experiences in Northern Italy', *BJSWS* 80-87.

[20] Cairns, H, Eden K.C, and Schorston, J. 'A Preliminary Report on the Treatment of Head Wounds with Penicillin. Investigation of War Wounds. Penicillin'. London: *War Office publication, A.M.D 7/90D/43,* 1943. During WW II, Major Schorstein spelt his name 'Schorston'.

[21] Connolly, R.C. 'The Management of the Untreated Brain Wound', *BJSWS* 168-172

[22] Schorstein, J. 'War Neurosurgery', *Manchester University Medical School Gazette,* 25 (1946), 58-67

[23] Small, J.M. and Turner, E.A. 'A Surgical Experience of 1200 Cases of Penetrating Brain Wounds in Battle, N.W. Europe', 1944-5, *BJSWS* 62-74; and Small, J.M, Turner, E.A, and Watt, A.C. 'The Management of Brain Wounds in the Forward Area', *BJSWS* 75-80.

[24] Johnson, R.T. 'Neurosurgery in Jungle Warfare', *Manchester University Medical School Gazette,* 25 (1946), 67-76.

[25] Cairns *BJSWS,* 11.

[26] Johnson, R.T, Dick R.C.S. 'Neurosurgery in the Eastern Theatre of War', *Lancet,* 2 (1945), 193-196; Johnson, R.T. 'Missile Wounds of the Head in the Burma Campaign', *BJSWS,* 172-177.

[27] Johnson, 1946, 68.

[28] Johnson, 1946, 71.

[29] Cairns, Eden, and Shoreston, 1943.

[30] For use of penicillin in WW2 see the Special Penicillin Issue of the *British Journal of Surgery,* 32 (1944-1945), 110-224.

[31] Cairns. *BJSWS,* 17

[32] Schurr, P.H. *So That was Life: A Biography of Sir Geoffrey Jefferson.* London: Royal Society of Medicine Press Limited, 1997.

[33] Rowbotham, G.F and Whalley N. 'A Series of Wounds of the Head from the Battle-Front of North-West Europe', *British Journal of Surgery,* (1947); War supplement No 1: 87-90.

Neuropathology in Germany During World War II: Julius Hallervorden (1882-1965) and the Nazi Programme of 'Euthanasia'

Summary: In Germany during World War II more than 120,000 handicapped children and adults were murdered for the convenience of the state. To gain scientific knowledge, the brains of many of these patients were examined by German neuropathologists. Some 698 of these specimens were examined in the Kaiser-Wilhelm-Institut für Hirnforchung in Berlin-Buch by Julius Hallervorden, whose career is reviewed together with that of his superior, Hugo Spatz. Hallervorden also oversaw the examination of cases of mental handicap by W-J Eiche at a laboratory at the Hospital Brandenburg-Gorden. Also in Berlin was Berthold Ostertag, neuropathologist at the Rudolf-Virchow-Hospital, who examined cases from the Children's Ward at Wiesengrund. Smaller but significant numbers of brains were examined in Munich, Heidelberg, Hamburg and Schleswig. Some brains of similar origin were examined in Vienna and in Lubliniecz. Jürgen Peiffer has estimated that German neuropathologists examined 2097 brains arising from the Nazi Programme of 'Euthanasia'.

Germany led the emergence of neuropathology as an academic discipline linked to psychiatry and, by the beginning of World War II, the bulk of published work in neuropathology was in German. The medical schools dominated German universities both in student numbers and in the seniority of medical staff. Psychiatry was the prominent specialty but from 1939 the international reputation of German psychiatry suffered from the link to the Nazi programme of 'euthanasia'[1] and ethnic murder.[2][3][4][5][6][7][8][9][10][11] German neuropathology was similarly tarnished, although few knew of its involvement, the subject of this article. Articles on this aspect of 'euthanasia' have appeared in German journals, notably by Jürgen Peiffer.[12][13][14][15] The evidence incriminates several neuropathologists but none exploited the scientific potential of 'euthanasia' more than Hallervorden. Whilst many doctors and several neuropathologists were involved in obtaining brains from the 'euthanasia' programme, Hallervorden was the most active participant and also among the most renowned in his speciality. His research, based on tissues of neurological cases, was materially assisted by his participation in 'euthanasia'.

Euthanasia and Nazi 'euthanasia'

The word euthanasia, from the Greek, means easy death but it has come to mean a planned death, where the time and method of dying is chosen by the subject for the relief of pain and suffering. But Nazi 'euthanasia' was the merciless murder of persons unwanted by the state. They were not in pain, they were not suffering, and only speed and convenience counted in the mode of death. In Germany the seeds of this movement which was linked to eugenics – the improvement of a population – antedate the Weimar Republic.[16] A minority held that the benefit to the state of the removal of unproductive lives outweighed humane considerations. In the aftermath of World War I when the population was near starvation, these views gained support in Germany but eugenics was also discussed in many countries including England and North America.[17 18 19] In Germany a publication in 1920 on 'The Ending of Lives Not Worth Living' by a Heidelberg doctor and a Leipzig lawyer was a typical product of this movement.[20] The justification of this solution of the problem of useless lives was stated. The right to live was earned by usefulness to the state. Ending of 'ballast lives' and 'empty husks' in mental institutions was the 'humane ' solution. This and earlier publications antedate the Nazi Party and Hitler, who adopted a movement already familiar to several relevant professions.[21]

Nazi 'Euthanasia' and Tiergartenstrasse 4, Berlin

A letter (translated) from Hitler, dated 1 September 1939 – the commencement of World War II – states:

> Reichsleiter Bouhler and Dr Brandt are entrusted with the responsibility of extending the rights of specially designated physicians, such that patients who are judged incurable after the most thorough review of their condition which is possible, can be granted mercy killing.[22]

This letter from Hitler begins the subject of this article but there is ample evidence of earlier planning of a state programme of 'euthanasia'.[23] The dating of this letter is significant. Hitler considered that the outbreak of war would diminish opposition to 'euthanasia' in Germany, and other countries would be less informed. Arising from this letter, *The Public Foundation for Medical and Institutional Care* [24] was formed in 1939, headed by Philipp Bouller (1899-1945) and Karl Brandt (1904-1947)[25] and from April 1940, was housed in a villa known as Tiergartenstrasse 4, Berlin (Figure 18.1). T4 became the abbreviation for the administrative centre, first for the programme of 'euthanasia' and later for the murder of millions of Jews, Gypsies, Poles, Russians and other unwanted persons in Germany and in the countries which Germany occupied. Many doctors, and especially psychiatrists worked for T4, which created and staffed the concentration camps and provided many camp commandants. T4 and all aspects of the

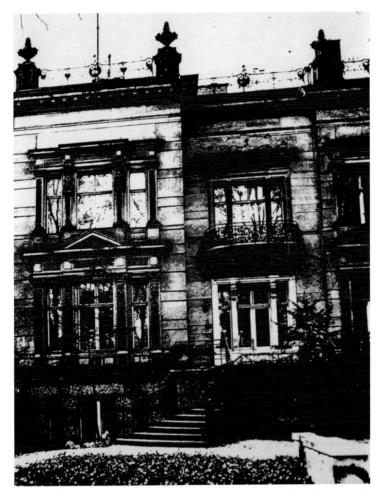

Figure 18.1 This inconspicuous villa at Tiergartenstrasse 4, Berlin was the administrative centre of the 'euthanasia' programme. The codename 'Aktion T-4' disguised its connection with KdF, the Chancellery of the Führer. The building did not survive World War II

'euthanasia' programme were staffed and administered by the Schutz-Staffel, the S.S. The 'euthanasia' programme itself caused about 275,000 deaths but has added importance as the beginning of the systematic murder of millions by the state.

Under the 'euthanasia' programme, inmates of state institutions, ill for five years or more and unable to work, were reported to T4. A completed questionnaire with name, age, race, next of kin, whether visited by relatives or friends, and whether supported financially, gave the information – all that was provided – to the consultant, usually a professor of psychiatry, who decided for or against execution.[26] Several organisations participated in the killing process. *The Realm's Work Committee of Institutions for Cure and Care* oversaw office procedures. Killing of children was organised by *The Realm's Committee for*

Scientific Approach to Severe Illness due to Heredity and Constitution. Patients were moved for killing by *The Charitable Transport Company for the Sick.* The *Charitable Foundation for Institutional Care* collected the costs of transport and killing from relatives, who were unaware of the movements and fate of their kin. Death certificates were falsely entered, with a fictitious cause of death and often a false date and place of death. Gassing by carbon monoxide was the original method of execution but other methods were developed such as the intravenous injection of petrol. Children were often starved to death. Adults and children suffered from a miscellany of neurological and psychiatric illnesses, examples being: mental sub-normality, poliomyelitis, multiple sclerosis, Parkinson's disease, pre-senile dementia, senile dementia, schizophrenia, and manic-depressive psychosis. Rarely did detailed notes accompanied a case but there were exceptions. An interesting mental condition might attract attention in which case the patient was examined carefully and necropsy and examination of the brain planned before death.

Julius Hallervorden

Hallervorden was born on 21 October 1882 in Allenberg, East Prussia (Figure 18.2).[27 28 29 30 31 32 33] His father, Dr Eugen Hallervorden then a psychiatrist in a local mental asylum, became Professor (Dozent) of Psychiatry at the University of Königsberg, to which town the family moved. Julius studied medicine at the university, obtaining his doctorate of medicine in 1909. He proceeded to Berlin where, for four years, he studied general medicine and psychiatry. In 1913 he was appointed to the psychiatric hospital of Landesberg an der Warthe where he worked for 33 years as a psychiatrist. He began the post-mortem study of the brains of his deceased patients, established his own laboratory and, self-taught, applied the recently introduced histological stains of neuropathology, notably the myelin stain of Carl Weigert (1845-1904) and the stain for neurone cell bodies of Franz Nissl (1860-1919). By presenting case studies to the Berlin Society for Psychiatry and Neurology, he attracted the notice of Walther Spielmeyer (1879-1935), who was the head of the new Neuropathology Institute in Munich and, in 1922, was to publish *Die Histopathologie des Nervensystems.*[34] In 1921 Spielmeyer perceiving a recruit to the discipline of neuropathology invited Hallervorden to his laboratory in Munich. There, Hallervorden met Hugo Spatz (1888-1969) (Figure 18.3) and together they studied the brain of a familial case of extra-pyramidal disorder. This brain, brought from Landesberg by Hallervorden, became the subject of the paper identifying Hallervorden-Spatz disease, now considered a neuroaxonal dystrophy.[35] Hallervorden and Spatz remained close friends and, when Spatz became director of the newly created Institute for Brian Research in Berlin, Hallervorden accompanied him.

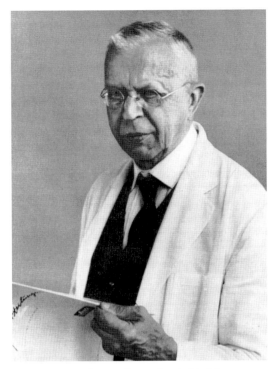

Figure 18.2 Julius Hallervorden in his laboratory.
From: *Archiv für Psychiatrie und Zeitscrift für Neurologie* (1965); 207: pp. 165-167

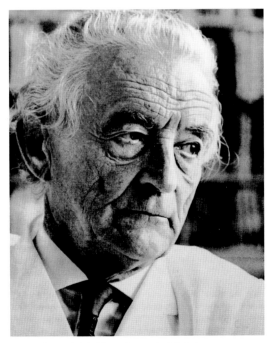

Figure 18.3 Hugo Spatz in his laboratory.
From: *Archiv für Psychiatrie und Nervenkrankheiten (*1969); 212: pp. 91-96

World War II and the Kaiser-Wilhelm Institut für Hirnforchung, Berlin-Buch (KWIH) (Figures 18.4 & 18.5)

Hugo Spatz was a neuroscientist of comparable stature to Hallervorden and, although six years younger, was Hallervorden's superior during WW II.[36][37] He succeeded Oscar Vogt as director of the KWIH in 1938 but also administered the Sections of Anatomy and of General Pathology. Hallervorden was in charge of neuropathology. World War II added many head injuries to neurology, neurosurgery, and neuropathology. The Air Force (Luftwaffe) carried out neurosurgery and most military head injuries came to the KWIH.[38] Spatz's rank was Oberfeldartz, and many of his staff held rank in the Luftwaffe. Hallervorden was a civilian consultant and directed the section dealing with army cases. He held the rank of Sonderfuhrer. Hundreds of cases of head injuries were examined and many scientific papers were published on these and on diseases of the brain. There was also experimental work.

The work of Hallervorden during World War II

There is direct evidence of the enthusiastic participation of Hallervorden in the 'euthanasia' programme.[39] His progress report to the *Deutsche Forchungsgemeinschaft*, dated 8 December 1942, states: 'In addition, during the course of this summer, I have been able to dissect 500 brains from feeble-minded individuals, and to prepare them for examination.' On 9 March 1944 he wrote to Professor Nitsche, then organising 'euthanasia': 'I have received 697 brains in all, including those which I took out myself in Brandenburg.' How Hallervorden viewed this participation in the programme was revealed when he was questioned by a member of the Office of the Chief of War Crimes at Nuremberg, United States Zone of Germany, 1946-7.[40] His interrogator was Major Leo Alexander, a psychiatrist in the US Army who had emigrated to North America from Vienna in 1933.[41][42][43][44][45] In June 1945, Alexander interviewed Hallervorden at Dillenberg in Hessen-Nassau where Hallervorden's section of special pathology was located in the Schloss Hotel. Despite these improvised quarters, to which the section had been evacuated in May 1944 because of the bombing of Berlin, Hallervorden's collection of more than 110,000 specimens from 2,800 cases was intact, accessible and catalogued. Major Alexander was shown the histological slides of selected cases with the clinical notes and the texts of published papers arising from the cases. Hallervorden's annual reports were available, showing the numbers of cases examined and the experiments performed. All the work was expertly examined and reported. Concerning the 'euthanasia' cases, Alexander quotes Hallervorden as saying:

> I heard that they were going to do that, and so I went up to them and told them 'Look here now, boys, if you are going to kill all these people, at least take the brains out so that the material could be utilised'. They asked me: 'How many

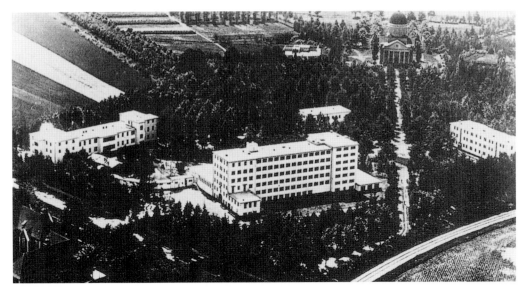

Figure 18.4 Aerial photograph of the Kaiser-Wilhelm-Institut für Hirnforchung in Berlin-Buch.

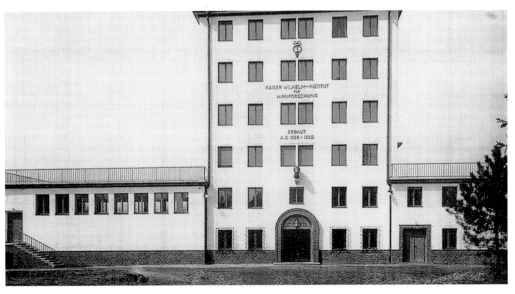

Figure 18.5 Frontal view from the East of the Kaiser-Wilhelm-Institut für Hirnforchung.

can you examine ?' and so I told them: 'an unlimited number – the more the better'. I gave them fixatives, jars and boxes, and instructions for removing and fixing the brains, and then they came bringing them in like a delivery van... There was wonderful material among those brains, beautiful mental-defectives, mal-formations and early infantile diseases. I accepted these brains of course. Where they came from and how they came to me was really none of my business.

Hallervorden planned the whole sequence of his scientific exploitation of 'euthanasia'. In 1940 he witnessed the killing of children by carbon monoxide at Brandenburg and at some necropsies he himself removed the brain.[46]   At Brandenburg, Dr Heinrich Bunke trained the staff and supervised the removal and fixation of the brains, techniques he had learnt during a four week period with Hallervorden at Berlin-Buch.[47]   Earlier, Major Alexander had questioned Spatz, then in Munich and still in charge of his section of anatomy and general pathology of the KWIH, formerly in Berlin.   Asked specifically about brains from the 'euthanasia' programme, Spatz (in Alexander's words):

> denied that he or any other member of his Institute [which would include Hallervorden] ever had received any. He added that the killing of the insane was done in deep secret, that nobody was supposed to know about it except SS personnel... that consequently no scientific institutions could be contacted in order to undertake neuropathological studies, and that thus invaluable pathologic material was lost and remained unutilised.[48]

It is significant that the versions given to Alexander by Hallervorden in Dillenberg and by Spatz in Munich differ widely. That of Hallervorden is credible: that of Spatz is not. Spatz, the director, could not be unaware of the brains arriving for study from these sources. The examination, by the elaborate techniques of neuropathology, of 697 brains would be an enormous addition to the other work of the KWIH. Recently, Jürgen Peiffer has examined surviving files and documents of 'euthanasia' cases in many neuropathological laboratories. His scrutiny of the Berlin-Buch files revealed 295 cases 'with certainty' and 403 cases 'with high probability' arising from 'euthanasia'. These figures agree almost exactly with those of Hallervorden.[49] Peiffer has examined the records of other laboratories in Berlin and elsewhere (see below) adding to the 698 cases in Berlin-Buch and giving a final conservative total of 2097 cases.

Neuropathology after World War II

German neuropathology recovered swiftly after World War II and, in classical neuropathology, remained ahead of the United Kingdom and North America, whose researchers, however, were developing and applying new techniques, such as electron microscopy, histochemistry and immunology. Young German neuroscientists were visiting the United Kingdom and North America for training: relatively few from North America and the UK went to visit Germany. The KWIH in Berlin was no more but neuropathology was supported in Cologne, Munich, and Frankfurt by the Max-Planck-Gessellschaft, the organisation that had replaced the Kaiser-Wilhelm-Gessellschaft. E.P. Richardson Junior, from the Massachusettes General Hospital, Boston, USA, visited Hallervorden in Giessen in 1955 and became his pupil for nearly six months. Richardson described Hallervorden in these words:

He was of a quiet, reserved nature, wholly devoted to science and to neuropathology, and, at the same time, warm, friendly, and an inspiring teacher. He was one of the last great figures of the classic period of German neuropathology.

Personal recollections of Hallervorden and Spatz

I met Hallervorden and Spatz many times when, in retirement, they were accommodated by Wilhelm Krücke in the Max-Planck-Institut für Hirnforschung, 46 Deutschorden Strasse, 6 Frankfurt a. M-Niederrad. Spatz was friendly and good company at luncheon and social occasions. His knowledge of neuropathology was immense, but his consuming interest then was comparative and developmental anatomy of the brain. In the two months I spent at Frankfurt, I found Hallervorden a helpful tutor. First acquaintance was disconcerting as his greeting was courteous but formal and it was clear that my visit was to be brief. But 'difficult to diagnose cases' from my Oxford laboratory quickly aroused his interest. Most were solved rapidly and he matched my cases with those from his own collections, but my cases of spinal cord softening puzzled him sufficiently to summon Spatz for a second opinion. These cases also interested Krücke, the director, and I presented them at the next meeting of the German Society at Würzburg when Krücke was president. The discussion of my cases was monopolised by contrary arguments from the floor by Hallervorden and Spatz.

From my first visit to Frankfurt in 1959, I was aware of a shadow cast in the Department of Neuropathology by the presence of Hallervorden. Neuropathology was housed with other disciplines of neuroscience in a magnificent new building and Krücke was the overall director. All the staff looked forward to an opening ceremony but this was postponed *sine die* as the publicity would be unwise when Hallervorden might still come to trial. The complicity of Spatz was never mentioned to me. Neither were brought to trial and the death of Hallervorden in 1965 and of Spatz in 1969 ended the possibility of any legal process. The obituaries of Hallervorden by Ule, Spatz, Krücke and Ostertag – his old colleagues –, and by van Bogaert of Antwerp, describe Hallervorden's scientific career at length, but make no mention of the subject of this article. Outside Germany, there was criticism. E.P. Richardson Junior, writing from Boston, USA in 1990, praised Hallervorden's achievements but added:

> It is impossible to escape the suspicion that some of the observations were made without appropriate considerations of the provenance of the material on which they were based.[50]

On the world stage there had been disquiet. In 1953, the preliminary organisers of the 5th International Congress of Neurology in Lisbon debated whether Hallervorden and Schaltenbrandt should be excluded. Georges Schaltenbrandt was accused of experiments on human subjects to prove or disprove whether an infectious agent could transmit multiple sclerosis. The culpability of Schaltenbrandt is outside the scope of this article but I can state that, when visiting his department, and his home in Würzburg and at subsequent meetings at conferences, it seemed that his wealth and fame had not been seriously diminished. Neuropathology held its first international conference in Rome in September 1952.[51] There were eleven German participants – the largest national group – with W. Scholtz, from Munich, as president. Hallervorden, then working at Giesen, gave the opening paper on the histopathology of the demyelinating diseases. Spatz, on the second day, spoke on brain damage from hypoxia and oligaemia and, on the fifth day, on Pick's disease. Spatz gave his two papers in French, a curious choice for a German speaking in Italy. Cecile and Osgar Vogt also spoke in French, but that was Cecile's native tongue.

Publications in Neuropathology after World War II

During and after the war Germany continued to dominate human neuropathology, as evidenced by the numerous papers published in German journals of pathology, psychiatry, neurology and neurosurgery. The magnitude of German neuropathology published after World War II, but based on earlier research, is seen in volume 13 of the *Handbuch der Speziellen Pathologischen Anatomie und Histologie*. Volume 13, entirely of neuropathology was edited by W Scholtz.[52] This 'volume 13' was subdivided into five 'volumes', but actually was completed in seven volumes. It provided a summary of human neuropathology, not available elsewhere and remains an outstanding source of reference and a monument to German neuropathology. These post-war publications in journals and books frequently identify human cases derived from the 'euthanasia' programme and we are indebted to Jürgen Peiffer for an analysis of this literature.[53]   The neuropathological laboratory can usually be identified, often the hospital of origin of a case and sometimes the name of a patient. It is helpful that important case reports are described more than once. Peiffer concluded that from Hallervorden's laboratory: 'twenty-five papers were published where we have to assume that some of the research was based on the victims of the 'euthanasia' programme'. Malformation of the brain was the speciality of Bertold Ostertag who was in Berlin at the same time as Hallervorden. Ostertag wrote the comprehensive account of this subject in one of the volumes of the Handbuch published in 1956. Examining his text shows that Ostertag drew extensively on cases from the 'euthanasia' programme. In no other subdivision of neuropathology was the correlation between case study and organised killing so clear.

From the Research Institute for Psychiatry in Munich, of which Scholtz was the director, eleven papers were published based on 'euthanasia' cases. Scholtz was the main author of the *Handbuch*. Other neuropathological centres in Germany[54] participated in this work and Peiffer's research has revealed the following numbers of cases: Lubliniecz, 209; Munich, 194; Heidelberg, 187; Hamburg, 49; and Schleswig, 21. These figures are of proven cases from the 'euthanasia' programme. Actual figures were probably higher and smaller numbers of cases were examined also in other laboratories. Peiffer has calculated that a total of 2097 brains were sent to laboratories from the 'euthanasia' programme.

Conclusions and Postscript

The evidence I have presented proves the active participation of Hallervorden in the scientific exploitation of 'euthanasia' cases. Without compulsion from his superiors, he sought this opportunity to advance the understanding of mental disease. Typical was his efficiency in pursuing his research and finding colleagues and technical staff despite the difficulties of wartime. He himself trained staff in the removal and preservation of brains at the place of execution, which he visited for this purpose. Even when Hallervorden moved from the ruins of Berlin to Dillenberg in Hessen-Nassau, his neuropathological collection of case notes, fixed tissues and histological slides was intact. It was still largely preserved when I visited the Max-Planck-Institut in Frankfurt in 1959 and on later visits. Hallervorden demonstrated cases to me and I was quite unaware of the controversial source of some of these. Hugo Spatz, overall director of the institute and the superior of Hallervorden, must also be held responsible. Spatz resorted to denial whereas Hallervorden openly revealed every record. Hallervorden believed that the ends – scientific discoveries – justified the means, a serious defect in the character of a distinguished scientist. Analysts of German medical research during World War II have suggested that much of the research, for example that on concentration camp inmates, was worthless, as such depraved scientists would not have produced reliable work. In the case material that came to Hallervorden, the care of the patient and the method of killing might have caused changes other than the condition that was being studied. For example, starvation often preceeded death. With this reservation, I cannot fault the accuracy of his neuropathological work. Finally, these crimes were committed by an outstanding world famous neuropathologist in a position of great authority and condoned by his superior, Hugo Spatz. Many of Hallervorden's colleagues followed his practice in obtaining research material, irrespective of an inexcusable source.

ACKNOWLEDGMENTS

I am indebted to the staff of the Radcliffe Science Library of the Bodleian Library, Oxford. The *Bundesarchiv, Koblenz* houses many of the manuscripts from which quotations have been reproduced. Professor Weindling of Oxford Brookes University provided me with a photostat copy of Alexander's typescript derived from the US National Archives. The pictures of Hallervorden and the KWIH were provided by

Sevda Kahraman of the *Institut für Geschichte de Medizin*, Ruprech-Karls-Universität, Heidelberg. The publications of Jürgen Peiffer and his personal communications were of especial value. Jürgen Peiffer died in December, 2006.

NOTES AND REFERENCES

[1] This 'euthanasia' did not benefit the subject. It was murder by the state to remove an unwanted person.

[2] Of the large literature on this subject, the nine books (refs 3-11) named below have been consulted.

[3] Aly. A.C. 'Nazi War Crimes of a Medical Nature'. In, *Ethics in Medicine: Historical. Perspectives and Contemporary Concerns*, edited by SJ Reiser, AJ Dyck & WJ Curran. Cambridge, Massachussets: MIT Press, 1971, 267-272.

[4] Müller-Hull B. *Tödlichen Wissenschaft*. Reinbeck bei Hamburg: Rowohlt Taschenbuch Verlag GmbH, 1984. English translation by GR Fraser as *Murderous Science*. Oxford: Oxford University Press, 1988. Page references are given from the reprint: New York: Cold Spring Harbor Laboratory Press, 1998. Müller-Hull gives the text of many primary sources.

[5] Proctor, R. *Racial Hygiene: Medicine under the Nazis*. Cambridge Mass: Harvard University Press, 1988. See chapter 7, 'The Destruction of 'Lives Not Worth Living', 177-222.

[6] Weindling, P. *Health, Race and German Politics between National Unification and Nazism 1870-1945*. Cambridge: Cambridge University Press, 1989.

[7] Kater, M.H. *Doctors under Hitler*. Chapel Hill and London: University of North Carolina Press, 1989.

[8] Annas, G.J. and Grodin, M.A, editors. *The Nazi doctors and the Nuremberg Code*. New York & Oxford: Oxford University Press, 1992.

[9] Caplan, A.L. *When Medicine went Mad*. Totowa, New Jersey: Humana Press, 1992.

[10] Deichman, U. *Biologen unter Hitler: Vertreibung, Karrieren, Forschung*. Frankfurt/Main: Campus Verlag, GmbH, 1992. English translation by Thomas Dunlap as *Biologists under Hitler*. Cambridge, Massachussets: Harvard University Press, 1966.

[11] Burleigh, M. *Death and Deliverance: Euthanasia in Germany 1900-1945*. Cambridge: Cambridge University Press, 1994 & Basingstoke and London: Pan Books, 2002.

[12] Peiffer, J. 'Zur Neurologie im 'Dritten Reich' und ihren Nachwirkungen', *Der Nervenartz*, 69 (1988), 728-733.

[13] Peiffer, J. 'Assessing neuropathogical research carried out on victims of the "Euthanasia" Programme', *Medizin Historisches Journal*, 34 (1999), 339-355.

[14] Peiffer J. 'Neuropathologische Forschung an 'Euthanasie' – Opfern in zwei Kaiser-Wilhelm Instituten'. In: *Geschichte der Kaiser-Wilhelm-Gesellschaft im Nationalsozialismus*, edited by D. Kaufmann. Gottingen: Wallstein Verlag, 2000, pp. 151-173.

[15] Peiffer, J. 'Phases in the post-war German reception of the "Euthanasia Program" (1939-1945) involving the killing of the mentally disabled and its exploitation by neuroscientists', *Journal of the History of the Neurosciences*, 15 (2006), 210-244. Peiffer's abundant references are a bibliography of the subject.

[16] The Racial Hygiene Society, founded in Berlin, was the first eugenics society (Weindling, *op. cit.* ref. 6): 141-142.

[17] In 1935, British Physicians formed the Voluntary Euthanasia Legalization Society, and a Bill was introduced to the House of Lords. *British Medical Journal*, 2 (1940), 881.

[18] Kennedy, F. 'The problem of Social Control of the Congenitally Defective: Education, Sterilization, and Euthanasia', *American Journal of Psychiatry*, 99 *(1942)*, 13-16.

[19] In England there was little support for eugenics. See Macnicol, J. 'Eugenics and the Campaign for Voluntary Sterilization in Britain between the Wars', *Social History of Medicine*, 2 (1989), 147-169.

[20] Binding, K and Hoche, A.E. *Die Freigabe der Vernichtung Lebensunwerten Lebens. Ihr Mass und Ihre Form.* Leipzig: F Meiner, 1920.

[21] This article describes the part played by psychiatrists and neuropathologists. Neuroanatomists and anthropologists were also active.

[22] *Bundesarchiv, Koblenz, R22-4209, p.1.* The document was backdated to 1 September 1939. The translated text is given in Muller-Hill, 1998 (*op. cit.* ref. 4): 43-44.

[23] Burleigh, 2002 (*op. cit.* ref 11): pp. 97-127.

[24] I give translations of the cynical titles of this organisation and those that follow.

[25] Bouhler committed suicide in 1945. Brandt was sentenced at Nuremberg and executed in 1947. Müller-Hill, 1998 (*op. cit.* ref. 4): 234.

[26] Processing was swift. One 'expert' examined 2109 questionnaires between 14 November and 1 December, 1940.

[27] There are many obituaries of Hallervorden – see below. Those of Ule, Spatz, Ostertag and Krücke avoided Hallervorden's part in the 'euthanasia' programme in which they themselves had participated. Van Bogaert denied the accusations. Richardson briefly mentioned the origin of some of Hallervorden's cases.

[28] Ule, G. 'Julius Hallervorden 1882-1965', *Archiv für Psychiatrie und Zeitscrift für Neurologie*, 207 (1965), 165-167.

[29] Spatz, H. 'Erinnerung an Julius Hallervorden (1882-1965)', *Der Nervenartz*, 37 (1966), 477-482.

[30] Krücke, W. 'Julius Hallervorden 1882-1965', *Acta Neuropathologica*, 6 (1966), 113-116.

[31] Ostertag, B. 'Julius Hallervorden, Sein Werken und sein Bedeutung fur die moderne Neuropathologie', *Die Medizinische Welt*, 4 (1967), 234-236.

[32] van Bogaert L. 'Julius Hallervorden (1882-1965)', *Journal of Neurological Science*, 5 (1967), 190-191.

[33] Richardson, E.P. junior. 'Julius Hallervorden'. In: Ashwal S. editor, *Founders of Child Neurology*, San Francisco: Norman Publishing, 1990, 506-512.

[34] Spielmeyer W. *Die Histopathologie des Nervensystems*, 1922, Berlin: J Springer.

[35] Hallervorden, J and Spatz, H. 1922. Eigenartige Erkrankung im extrapyramidalen System mit besonderer Beteiligung des Globus Pallidus und der Substantia Nigra, *Zeitschrift für Neurologie und Psychiatrie*, 79 (1922), 254-302.

[36] Scholtz W. 'Hugo Spatz 1888-1969', *Archiv Psychiatrie Nervenkrankheit*, 212 (1969), 91-96.

[37] van Bogaert L. Hugo Spatz (1888-1969). In: *The Founders of Neurology*. Editors W

Haymaker and F Schiller, 2nd edition, Springfield, Illinois: Charles C Thomas, 1970, 369-375.

[38] Decompression injuries were directed to Professor Buchner at Freiburg.

[39] Müller Hill (*op. cit.* ref. 4): p. 18.

[40] Leo Alexander's report is entitled *Neuropathology and Neurophysiology, including Electro-encephalography, in Wartime Germany*. The 65 pages of typescript are held in the National Archives, Washington DC, Document L-170.

[41] Alexander subsequently wrote several articles based on his investigations in occupied Germany immediately after World War 2. Four (refs. 42-45) are cited below.

[42] Alexander, L. 'War Crimes: their social-psychological aspects', *American Journal of Psychiatry,* 105 (1948), 170-177.

[43] Alexander, L. 'Sociopsychological structure of the SS: psychiatric report of the Nuremberg trials for war crimes', *Archives of Neurology & Psychiatry,* 59 (1948), 622-634.

[44] Alexander L. 'War crimes and their motivation: socio-psychological structure of SS and criminalisation of society', *Journal of Criminal Law & Criminology,* 39 (1948), 298-326.

[45] Alexander, L. 'Medical Science under Dictatorship', *New England Journal of Medicine,* 241 (1949), 39-47.

[46] Muller-Hill (*op. cit.* ref. 4): 21.

[47] Dr Bunke's statement at his trial is preserved at Frankfurt/Main Hessisches Haupstaatsarchiv, Wiesbaden, *Sign. GenStA Frankfurt Js 15/61.*

[48] Although the activities of the SS in T4 were secret, I consider Spatz's denial implausible.

[49] Peiffer 1999 (*op. cit.* ref. 13): 345.

[50] Richardson (*op. cit.* ref. 32): 511.

[51] *Proceedings of the First International Conference of Neuropathology, Rome, September 8-13 1952.* Torino: Rosenberg & Sellier, 1953.

[52] Scholtz, W. Editor of Nervensystems, volume 13 (5 volumes in 7 parts) of *Handbuch der Spezielle Pathologische Anatomie und Histologie.* Berlin, Gôttinigen, Heidelberg: Springer. Publication of the volume 13 began in 1957.

[53] Peiffer (*op. cit.* ref. 13) (1999) 348-350.

[54] and Vienna

INDEX